AF324722

Lean and Green Recipes for Beginners

Quick and Easy Recipes to Stay Fit and Boost Your Metabolism

Linda Carey

Table of contents

Green Buddha Bowl

Prep Time: 15 minutes.

Cook Time: 0 minutes.

Serves: 2

Ingredients:

- 1 tablespoon olive oil
- 1 lb brussels sprouts, trimmed and halved
- Salt and black pepper, to taste
- 2 cups cooked quinoa
- 1 cup red apple, chopped
- ¼ cup pepitas
- 1 avocado, sliced
- 1 ½ cups arugula
- ½ cup of mayo
- ¾ cup plain Greek yogurt
- 1 teaspoon ground mustard
- ¼ cup Pompeian White Balsamic Vinegar
- ½ teaspoon salt
- 1 tablespoon fresh basil, chopped
- 1 garlic clove, minced

Preparation:

1. Mix quinoa with apple and the rest of the ingredients in a salad bowl.

2. Serve.

Serving Suggestion: Serve the bowl with spaghetti squash.

Variation Tip: Add some edamame beans to the bowl.

Nutritional Information Per Serving:

Calories 318 | Fat 15.7g |Sodium 124mg | Carbs 27g | Fiber 0.1g | Sugar 0.3g | Protein 4.9g

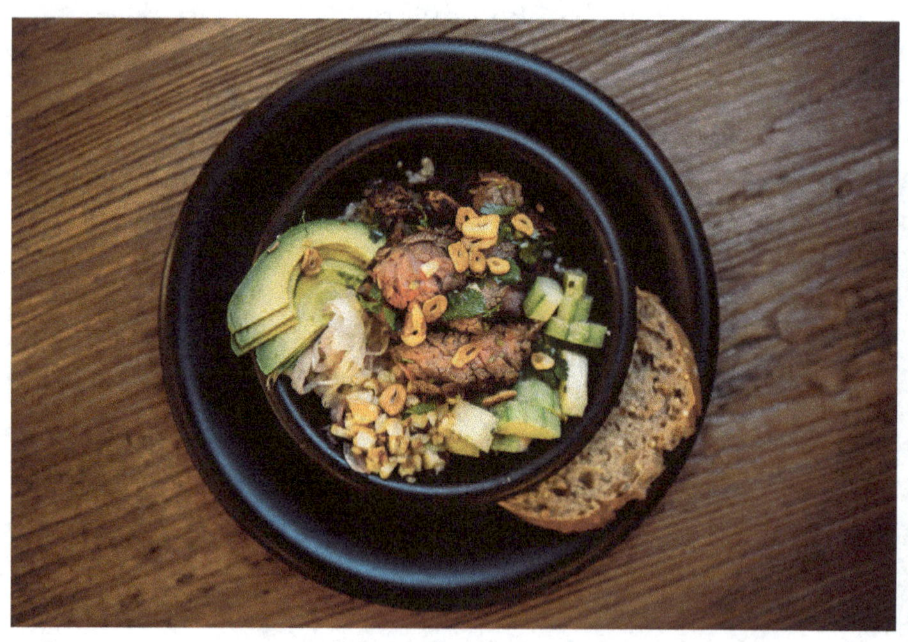

Lean Mean Soup

Prep Time: 15 minutes.

Cook Time: 30 minutes.

Serves: 6

Ingredients:

- 1/2 head cabbage, chopped
- 3 cups broccoli, chopped
- 1 cup carrots, diced
- 8 stalks celery, diced
- 1 cup onion, diced
- 1 cup radishes, chopped
- 1/2 cup yellow pepper, diced
- 1/2 cup red pepper, diced
- 1/2 cup orange pepper, diced
- 2 tablespoons garlic, minced
- 1 -6 ounce can tomato paste
- 2 -14-ounce cans diced tomatoes with green chiles, undrained
- 6 1/2 cups water
- 1 teaspoon dried parsley
- 1 teaspoon dried oregano
- 1 teaspoon turmeric
- 1/2 cup kale
- Salt and black pepper, to taste

Preparation:

1.   Add all the green soup ingredients to a cooking pot.
2.   Cook for 30 minutes on low heat until veggies are soft.
3.   Serve warm.

Serving Suggestion: Serve the soup with cauliflower rice.

Variation Tip: Add broccoli florets to the soup as well.

Nutritional Information Per Serving:

Calories 114 | Fat 2.2g |Sodium 276mg | Carbs 27.7g | Fiber 0.9g | Sugar 1.4g | Protein 8.8g

Spaghetti Squash

Prep Time: 15 minutes.

Cook Time: 45 minutes.

Serves: 4

Ingredients:

- 1 spaghetti squash
- 1 pinch black pepper
- 1 tablespoon olive oil
- 1 tablespoon Pecorino Romano, shredded

Preparation:

1. At 425 degrees F, preheat your oven.
2. Cut the spaghetti squash in half, remove its seeds and place in a baking sheet.
3. Drizzle black pepper, and olive oil on top, then bake for 45 minutes.
4. Scrap the squash flesh with a fork and add to the serving plate.
5. Drizzle pecorino Romano on top.
6. Serve.

Serving Suggestion: Serve the squash with roasted mushrooms.

Variation Tip: Add lemon zest and lemon juice for better taste.

Nutritional Information Per Serving:

Calories 324 | Fat 5g |Sodium 432mg | Carbs 13.1g | Fiber 0.3g | Sugar 1g | Protein 5.7g

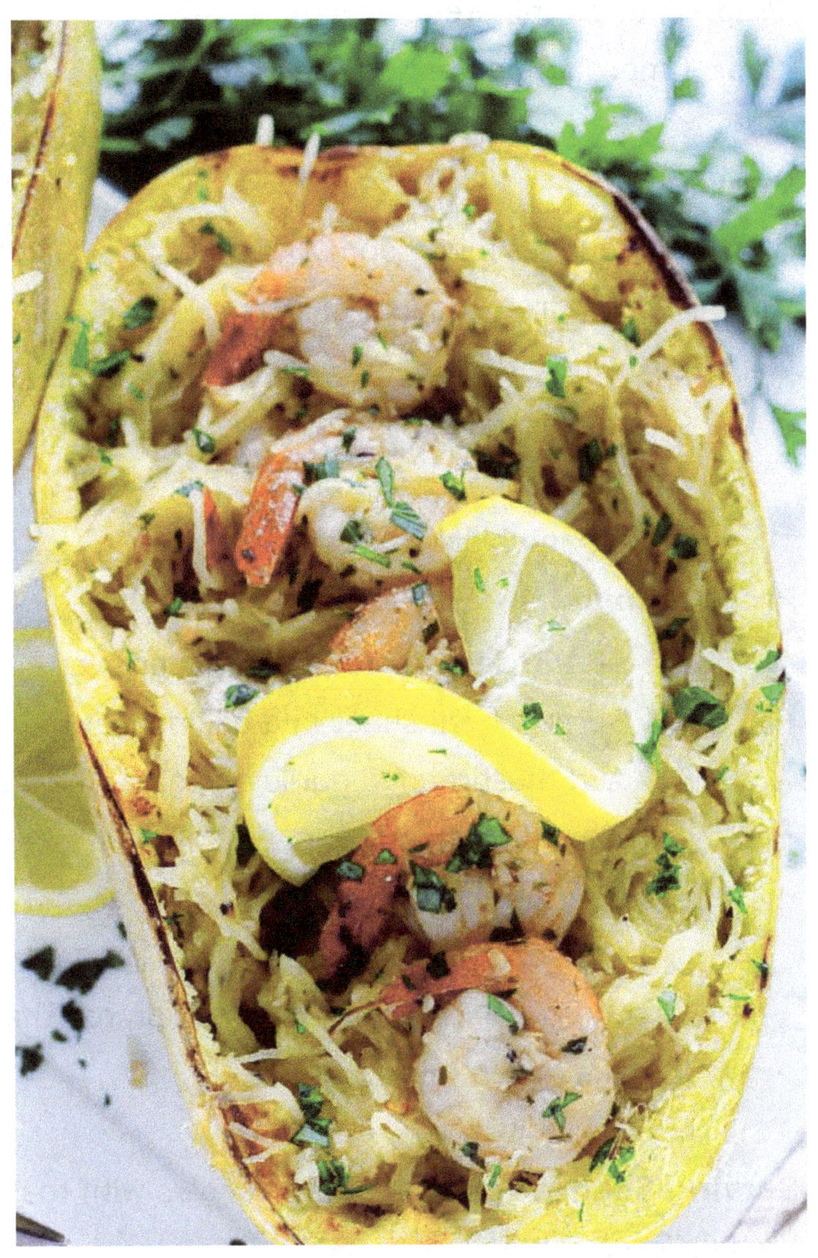

Roasted Green Beans and Mushrooms

Prep Time: 15 minutes.

Cook Time: 25 minutes.

Serves: 4

Ingredients:

- 8 ounces mushrooms, cleaned and halved
- 1 lb. green beans, halved
- 8 whole garlic cloves, halved
- 2 tablespoons olive oil
- 1 tablespoon balsamic vinegar
- Salt and black pepper, to taste

Preparation:

1. At 450 degrees F, preheat your oven.
2. Spread a foil sheet in a baking tray.
3. Add mushrooms, garlic and green beans to the baking sheet.
4. Mix balsamic vinegar with olive oil in a small bowl and pour over the veggies.
5. Drizzle black pepper and salt on top then bake for 25 minutes.
6. Serve warm.

Serving Suggestion: Serve the veggies with toasted bread slices.

Variation Tip: Add boiled zucchini pasta to the mixture.

Nutritional Information Per Serving:

Calories 136 | Fat 10g |Sodium 249mg | Carbs 8g | Fiber 2g | Sugar 3g | Protein 4g

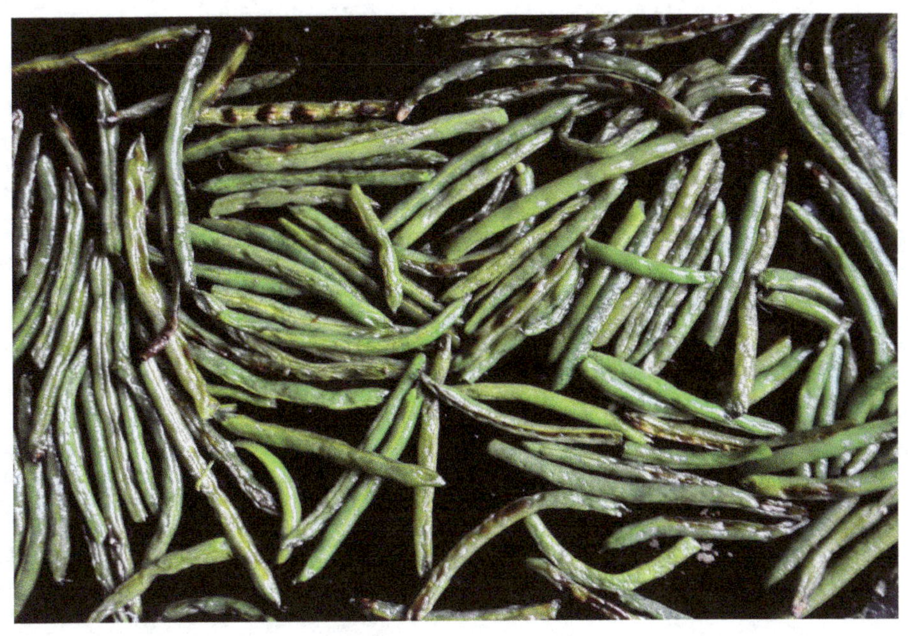

Mexican Cauliflower Rice

Prep Time: 15 minutes.

Cook Time: 14 minutes.

Serves: 4

Ingredients:

- 1 head cauliflower, riced
- 1 tablespoon olive oil
- 1 medium white onion, diced
- 2 garlic cloves, minced
- 1 jalapeno, seeded and minced
- 3 tablespoons tomato paste
- 1 teaspoon of sea salt
- 1 teaspoon cumin
- 1/2 teaspoon paprika
- 3 tablespoons fresh cilantro, chopped
- 1 tablespoon lime juice

Preparation:

1. Grate the cauliflower in a food processor.
2. Sauté onion with oil in a skillet over medium-high heat for 6 minutes.
3. Stir in jalapeno and garlic, then sauté for 2 minutes.
4. Add paprika, cumin, salt, and tomato paste, then sauté for 1 minute.

5. Stir in cauliflower rice and the rest of the ingredients and cook for 5 minutes.

6. Add cilantro and lime juice in the top.

7. Serve.

Serving Suggestion: Serve the rice with roasted veggies on the side.

Variation Tip: Add canned corn to the rice.

Nutritional Information Per Serving:

 Calories 351 | Fat 19g |Sodium 412mg | Carbs 43g | Fiber 0.3g | Sugar 1g | Protein 23g

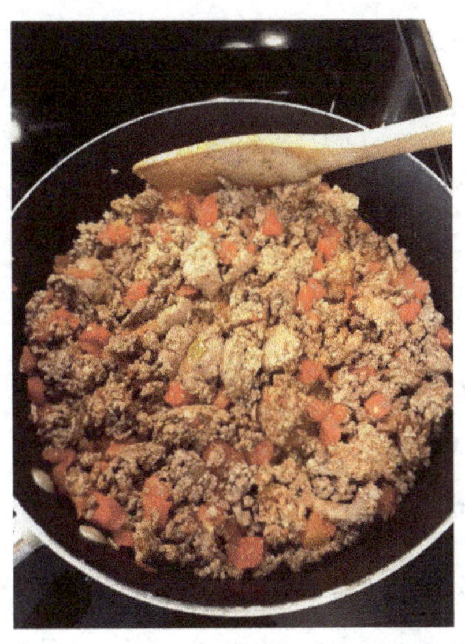

Sheet Pan Chicken

Prep Time: 15 minutes.

Cook Time: 18 minutes.

Serves: 4

Ingredients:

- 1 ¾ pounds boneless chicken breasts, diced
- Salt, to taste
- 1 pound broccoli crowns
- 1 medium red bell pepper
- 2 tablespoons olive oil
- ¼ cup peanut butter
- 1 tablespoon tamari
- 1 tablespoon rice vinegar
- 1 tablespoon honey
- juice from ½ lime
- 3 tablespoons water
- 1 pinch of salt
- Sesame seeds
- Sliced green onions

Preparation:

1. At 425 degrees F, preheat your oven.
2. Layer 2 baking sheets with wax paper and grease with cooking spray.

3. Toss chicken, veggies and all the ingredients in a large bowl.

4. Divide this mixture in the prepared baking seet.

5. Bake the mixture for 18 minutes in the oven.

6. Garnis whti sesame seeds and green onions.

7. Serve warm.

Serving Suggestion: Serve the chicken with a kale salad on the side.

Variation Tip: Coat the chicken with coconut shreds for a crispy texture.

Nutritional Information Per Serving:

Calories 384 | Fat 15g |Sodium 587mg | Carbs 8g | Fiber 1g | Sugar 5g | Protein 20g

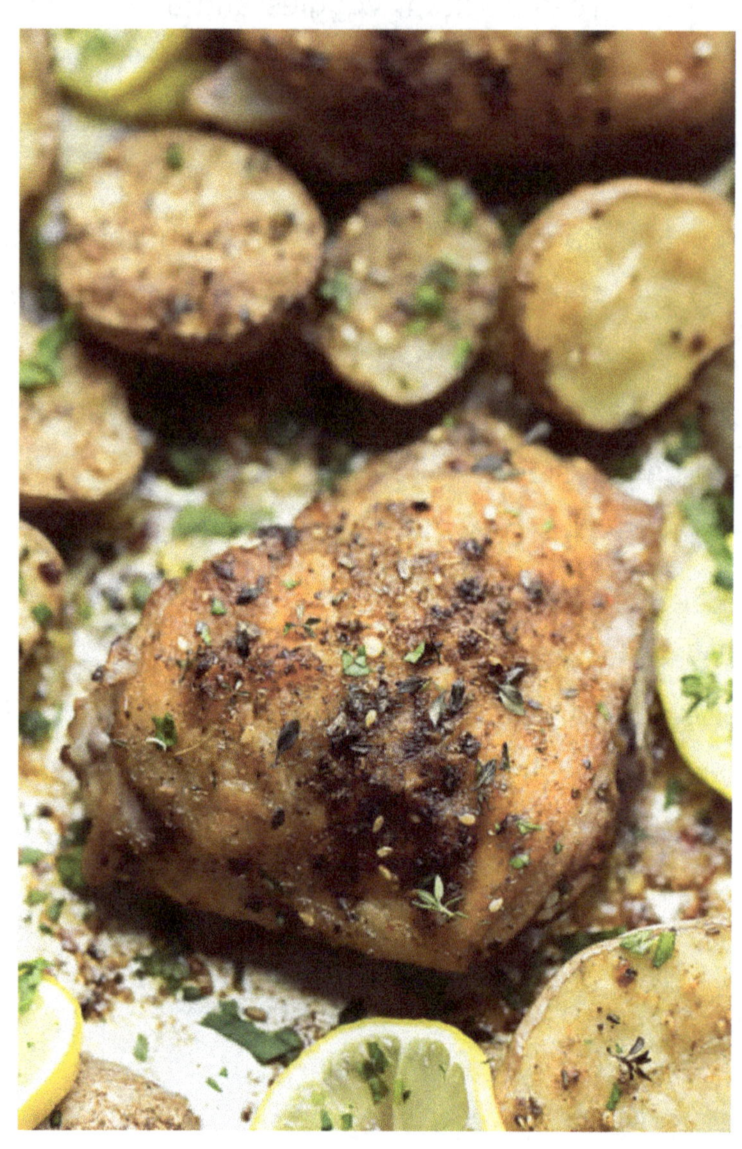

Green Chicken Casserole

Prep Time: 15 minutes.

Cook Time: 25 minutes.

Serves: 6

Ingredients:

- 6 whole wheat tortillas
- 1 (15-oz) can white beans
- 1 (12-oz) bag cheese mexican blend, shredded
- 1 cup monterey jack cheese, shredded
- 1 (24-oz) jar salsa verde
- 2 (4-oz) cans of green hatch chiles
- 1 cup shredded salsa chicken
- 1 tablespoon dried oregano

TOPPINGS

- Greek Yogurt
- Guacamole
- Hot sauce
- Fresh cilantro

Preparation:

1. At 375 degrees F, preheat your oven.

2. Spread four tortilla halves in a 9x13 inches baking dish.

3. Top the tortillas with salsa verde to cover.

4. Mix beans with chile mixture and chicken in a bowl.

5. Sprread half of this mixture over the salsa verde.

6. Repeat the layers and top with cheese.

7. Bake for 25 mminutes in the oven at 375 degrees F.

8. Serve warm.

Serving Suggestion: Serve the casserole with roasted green beans.

Variation Tip : Add some sliced onion and spring onion to the casserole.

Nutritional Information Per Serving:

Calories 335 | Fat 5g |Sodium 422mg | Carbs 16g | Fiber 0g | Sugar 1g | Protein 25g

Broccoli Chicken Casserole

Prep Time: 15 minutes.

Cook Time: 20 minutes.

Serves: 4

Ingredients:

- 2 pounds boneless chicken breasts
- 1 tablespoon olive oil
- 2 10-ounce bags frozen cauliflower rice
- 1 (16-ounce) bag frozen broccoli cuts
- 2 large eggs, whisked
- 3 cups mozzarella cheese, shredded
- 2 teaspoons salt
- 2 teaspoons garlic powder
- 2 teaspoons onion powder
- 2 tablespoons butter, melted
- 1 cup Italian blend cheese, shredded

Preparation:

1. At 400 degrees F, preheat your oven.
2. Grease a baking dish with cooking spray.
3. Rub the chicken with oil, black pepper and salt then place in the baking sheet.
4. Bake the chicken breasts for 20 minutes.
5. Cook the cauliflower rice and broccoli as per the package's instructions.

6. Cut the baked chicken into cubes.

7. Mix chicken with rest of the ingredients in a bowl.

8. Spread this mixture in the baking dish and bake for 50 minutes in the oven.

9. Serve warm.

Serving Suggestion: Serve the casserole with roasted veggies.

Variation Tip: Add chopped carrots to the casserole.

Nutritional Information Per Serving:

Calories 369 | Fat 14g |Sodium 442mg | Carbs 13.3g | Fiber 0.4g | Sugar 2g | Protein 32.3g

Chicken with Green Beans

Prep Time: 15 minutes.

Cook Time: 11 minutes.

Serves: 4

Ingredients:

- 1 pound chicken breast cutlets
- 1 teaspoon salt, divided
- ½ teaspoon black pepper
- 2 tablespoons olive oil
- 6 cups green beans, trimmed
- 4 garlic cloves, sliced
- 1 teaspoon lemon zest, grated
- 1 teaspoon fresh thyme, chopped
- ¼ cup chicken broth
- ¼ cup dry white wine
- 1 tablespoon lemon juice
- ¼ cup pine nuts, toasted
- Lemon wedges for garnish

Preparation:

1. Season the chicken with black pepper, oil and salt.
2. Sear the chicken cutlets for 4 minutes per side in a skillet.

3. Sautte green beans with salt, oil and black pepper in a pan for 2 minutes.

4. Stir in wine, broth a nd lemon juie.

5. Cook for 1 minute then add chicken.

6. Garnish with pine nuts, lemon wedges and thyme.

7. Serve warm.

Serving Suggestion: Serve the chicken with fresh cucumber and couscous salad.

Variation Tip: Add some green peas to the mixture.

Nutritional Information Per Serving:

Calories 453 | Fat 2.4g |Sodium 216mg | Carbs 18g | Fiber 2.3g | Sugar 1.2g | Protein 23.2g

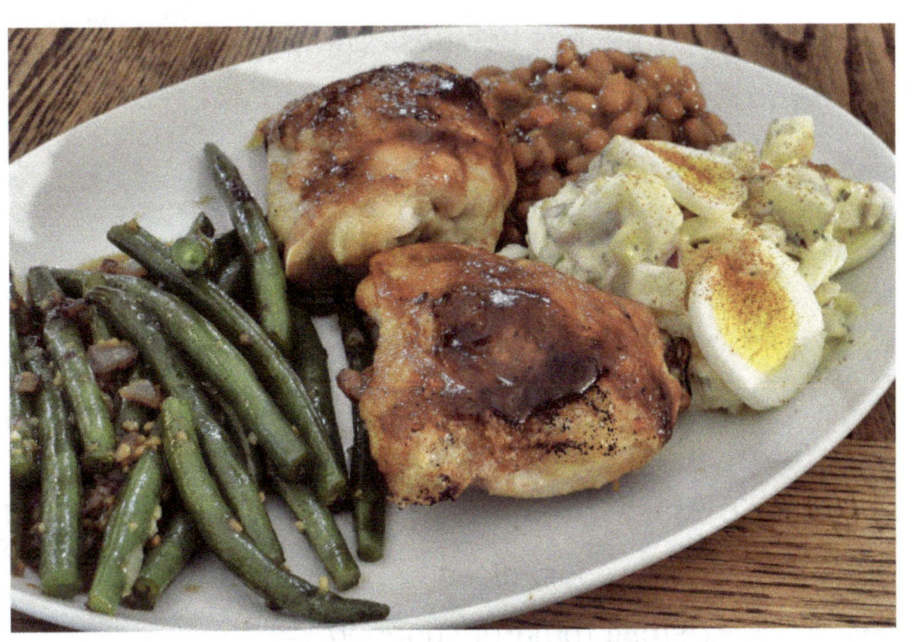

Chicken with Avocado Salsa

Prep Time: 15 minutes.

Cook Time: 42 minutes.

Serves: 2

Ingredients:

- 1 ½ pounds boneless chicken breasts

Marinade

- 2 garlic cloves, minced
- 3 tablespoons olive oil
- ¼ cup cilantro, chopped
- Juice of 1 lime
- ½ teaspoons salt
- ¼ teaspoons black pepper

Avocado Salsa

- 2 avocados, diced
- 2 small tomato, chopped
- ¼ cup red onion, chopped
- 1 jalapeno, deseeded and chopped
- 1/4 cup cilantro, chopped
- Juice of 1 lime
- Black pepper and salt to taste

Preparation:

1.   Mix all the marinade ingredients in a bowl.

2.   Pound and flatten each chicken breast into ¼ inch thickness.

3.   Add this chicken to the marinade, mix well, cover and refrigerate for 30 minutes.

4.   Grill the chicken for 6 minutes per side in a preheated grill.

5.   Serve the chicken with the avocado salsa.

6.   Mix all the avocado salsa ingredients in a bowl.

7.   Enjoy.

Serving Suggestion: Serve the chicken with cauliflower rice.

Variation Tip: Add dried herbs to the mixture for seasoning.

Nutritional Information Per Serving:

Calories 331 | Fat 20g |Sodium 941mg | Carbs 30g | Fiber 0.9g | Sugar 1.4g | Protein 24.6g

Cheddar Turkey Burgers

Prep Time: 15 minutes.

Cook Time: 14 minutes.

Serves: 4

Ingredients:

- 1 lb lean ground turkey
- 1 (1 ounce) envelope dry ranch dressing
- 1 cup cheddar cheese, shredded
- 1/4 cup green onion, chopped

Preparation:

1. Mix turkey ground with ranch dressing, cheese and green onion in a bowl.
2. Make six patties out of this mixture.
3. Sear each patty in a skillet for 7 minutes per side.
4. Serve warm.

Serving Suggestion: Serve the burgers with fresh herbs on top.

Variation Tip: Add some chopped bell pepper to the patties.

Nutritional Information Per Serving:

Calories 332 | Fat 18g |Sodium 611mg | Carbs 13.3g | Fiber 0g | Sugar g4 | Protein 38g

Turkey Taco Soup

Prep Time: 15 minutes.

Cook Time: 45 minutes.

Serves: 6

Ingredients:

- 1 ½ lbs. lean ground turkey
- 1 onion, diced
- 1 (1 ¼ ounces) package taco seasoning
- 1 (1 ounce) package ranch dressing seasoning
- 1 (14oz) can chicken broth
- 1 (4 ounces) can diced green chiles
- 1 (15 ½ ounces) can whole kernel corn
- 1 (15 ½ ounces)can pinto beans
- 1 (15 ounces) can refried beans
- 1 (14 ½ ounces) can diced tomatoes with green chiles
- 1 (14 ½ ounces) can mexican diced tomatoes

Preparation:

1. Saute onion and turkey in a skillet until golden brown.
2. Stir in rest of the ingredients and cook for 45 minutes.
3. Serve warm.

Serving Suggestion: Serve the soup with toasted bread slices.

Variation Tip: Add zucchini noodles to the soup.

Nutritional Information Per Serving:

Calories 354 | Fat 25g |Sodium 412mg | Carbs 22.3g | Fiber 0.2g | Sugar 1g | Protein 28.3g

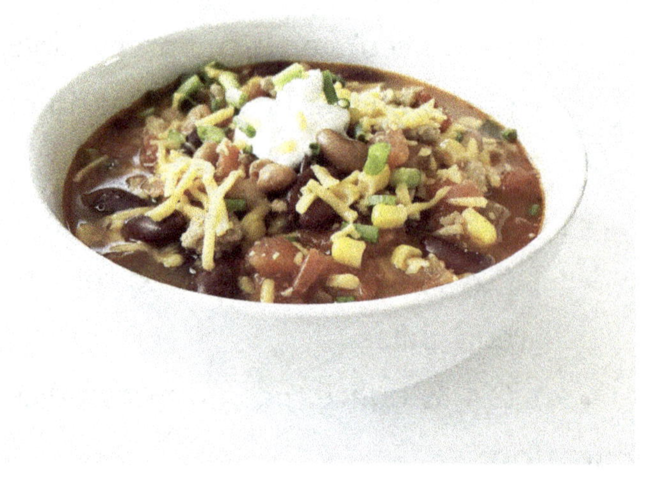

Chicken Zucchini

Prep Time: 15 minutes.

 Cook Time: 30 minutes.

Serves: 4

Ingredients:

- 4 pieces of chicken breast
- 1 cup Zucchini, chopped
- 2 tablespoons shredded cheese
- 1 raw onion, chopped
- Salt, to taste
- Black pepper, to taste
- Oregano, to taste

Preparation:

1. At 450 degrees F, preheat your oven.
2. Place the chicken breast in a baking pan and drizzle oregano, black pepper and salt on top.
3. Drizzle cheese on top and cover the chicken with zucchini slices.
4. Bake this chicken for 30 minutes in the oven.
5. Serve warm.

Serving Suggestion: Serve the chicken with white rice or sweet potato salad.

Variation Tip: Add some zucchini noodles to the chicken.

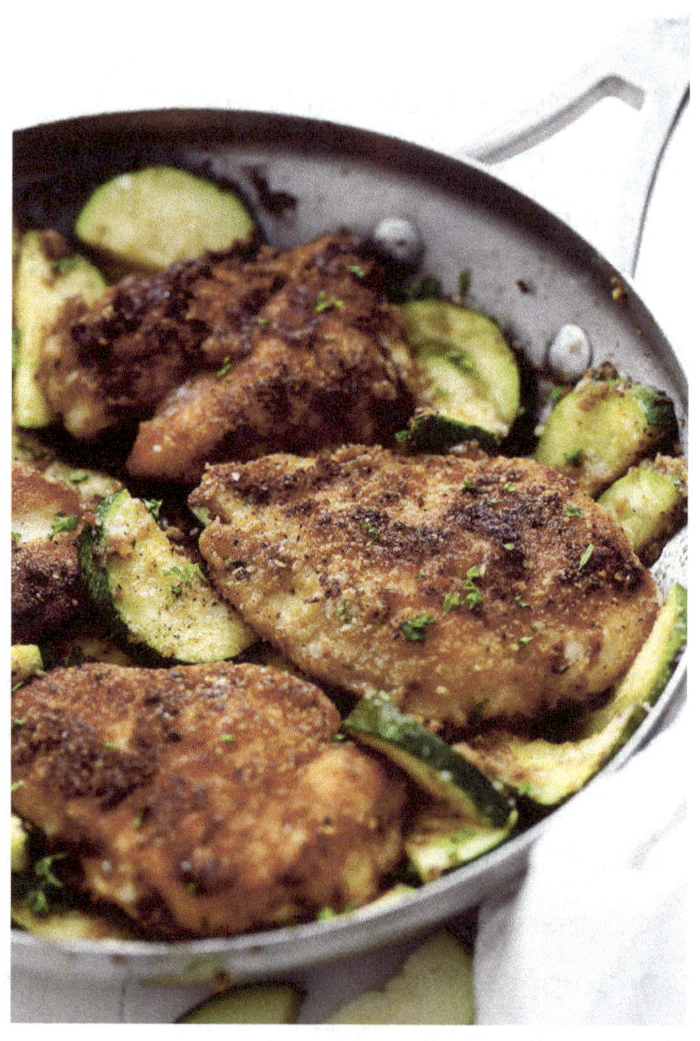

Turkey Shepherd's Pie

Prep Time: 15 minutes.

Cook Time: 30 minutes.

Serves: 4

Ingredients:

- 12 ounces lean ground turkey
- 2 cups cooked potatoes, mashed
- 1 cup frozen corn
- 1/2 cup tomatoes, diced
- 1/2 cup carrots, diced
- 1/2 cup zucchini, diced
- 1/4 cup onions, chopped
- 3 teaspoons garlic, minced
- salt and black pepper, to taste

Preparation:

1. Sauté turkey with black pepper, salt, garlic, carrots, and onion in a skillet until golden brown.
2. Spread the turkey in a 9x12 inch baking pan.
3. Top it with tomatoes, zucchini, carrots, garlic and onion.
4. Add frozen corn and mashed potatoes on top.

5. Bake this casserole for 20 minutes in the oven at 350 degrees F.

6. Serve warm.

Serving Suggestion: Serve the pie with avocado tomato salad.

Variation Tip: Add boiled peas to the pie.

Nutritional Information Per Serving:

Calories 352 | Fat 14g |Sodium 220mg | Carbs 16g | Fiber 0.2g | Sugar 1g | Protein 26g

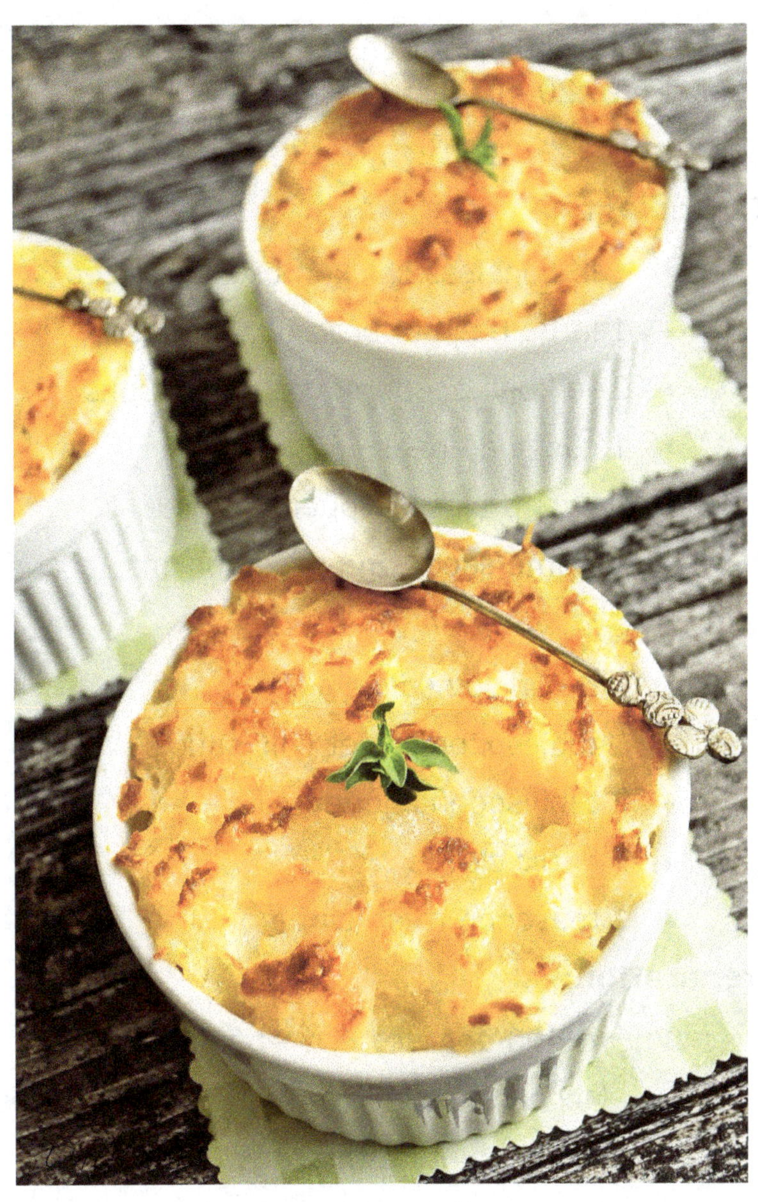

Sesame Chicken

Prep Time: 15 minutes.

Cook Time: 20 minutes.

Serves: 2

Ingredients:

- 1 lb boneless chicken breasts, diced
- 1 large head of broccoli, chopped
- 2 red bell peppers, cut into chunks
- 1 cup snap peas
- Salt and black pepper, to taste
- Sesame seeds and green onions

Sauce:

- 1/4 cup soy sauce
- 1 tablespoon sweet chili sauce
- 2 tablespoons honey
- 2 garlic cloves
- 1 teaspoon fresh ginger

Preparation:

1. At 400 degrees F, preheat your oven.
2. Mix all the sauce ingredients in a saucepan and cook until it thickens.
3. Remove the sauce from the heat and allow the sauce to cool.

4.   Spread the veggies and chicken in a greased baking sheet.

5.   Drizzle sauce over the mixture and mix well.

6.   Bake the mixture for 20 minutes in the oven.

7.   Garnish with sesame seeds.

8.   Serve warm.

Serving Suggestion: Serve the chicken with toasted bread on the side.

Variation Tip: Add some canned corn to the meal.

Nutritional Information Per Serving:

Calories 334 | Fat 16g |Sodium 462mg | Carbs 31g | Fiber 0.4g | Sugar 3g | Protein 25.3g

Turkey Broccoli

Prep Time: 15 minutes.

Cook Time: 20 minutes.

Serves: 4

Ingredients:

- 1 tablesepoon Dijon mustard
- 1 tablespoon whole grain mustard
- 1 cup chicken broth
- 4 teaspoons roasted garlic oil
- 4 cups broccoli florets
- 1 tablespoon garlic gusto seasoning
- 1½ lb boneless turkey breasts, diced
- 1 pinch dash of desperation seasoning

Preparation:

1. Mix broth with mustard in a bowl.
2. Saute broccoli with oil and garlic gusto in a skillet for 2 minutes.
3. Transfer the broccoli to a bowl.
4. Sear the turkey bites in the same pan for 5 minutes per side.
5. Reduce heat, and stir in mustard mixture and broccoli.
6. Cover and cook for 7 minutes on a simmer.
7. Serve warm.

Serving Suggestion: Serve the chicken with a spinach salad.

Variation Tip: Add chopped green beans to the mixture.

Nutritional Information Per Serving:

 Calories 388 | Fat 8g |Sodium 339mg | Carbs 8g | Fiber 1g | Sugar 2g | Protein 33g

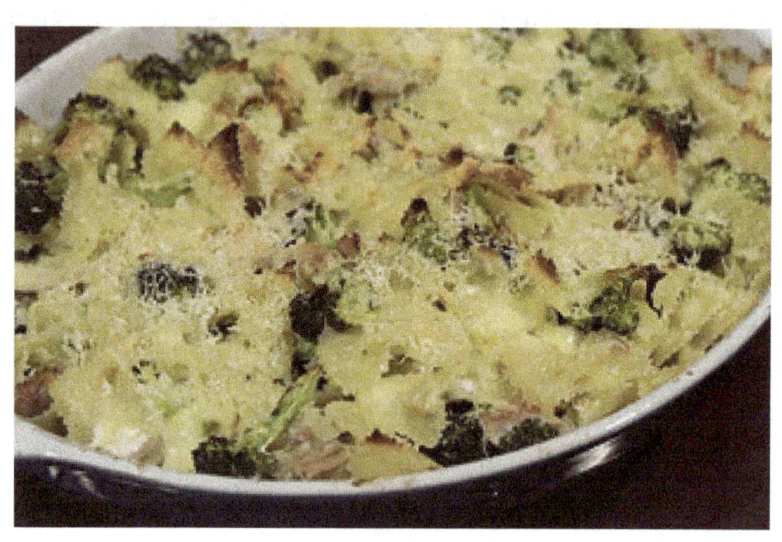

Chicken Piccata

Prep Time: 15 minutes.

Cook Time: 10 minutes.

Serves: 8

Ingredients:

- 8 boneless chicken breast halves
- 3 teaspoons olive oil
- 2 tablespoons butter
- 1/2 cup all-purpose flour
- 1/2 cup Parmesan cheese, grated
- 1/2 cup egg
- 1/2 teaspoon salt
- 2 tablespoons 1/4 cup dry white wine
- 1/4 cup parsley minced
- 1/8 teaspoon hot pepper sauce
- 5 tablespoons lemon juice
- 3 garlic cloves, minced

Preparation:

1. Pound and flatten each chicken piece.
2. Beat egg with hot pepper sauce, garlic, and 2 tablespoons lemon juice in a bowl.
3. Mix flour with salt, parsley, and Parmesan cheese in a bowl.

4. First coat the chicken with the flour mixture then dip in the egg mixture and coat again with the flour mixture.

5. Place the coated chicken a greased skillet and cook for 5 minutes per side.

6. Mix lemon juice, melted butter and remaining wine in a saucepan and boil.

7. Drizzle this sauce over the chicken.

8. Serve warm.

Serving Suggestion: Serve the chicken with a fresh crouton's salad.

Variation Tip: Add a drizzle of cheese on top.

Nutritional Information Per Serving:

Calories 300 | Fat 2g |Sodium 374mg | Carbs 30g | Fiber 6g | Sugar 3g | Protein 32g

Baked Chicken Stuffed

Prep Time: 15 minutes.

Cook Time: 22 minutes.

Serves: 4

Ingredients:

- 4 chicken breast halves
- 4 ounces baby bella mushrooms
- 1/4 cup onion, chopped
- 1/2 teaspoon ground thyme
- 1/2 teaspoon salt
- 1/4 cup mozzarella cheese, shredded

Preparation:

1. At 350 degrees F, preheat your oven.
2. Layer a 9x13 inches baking dish with cooking oil.
3. Saute mushrooms, onions, salt and thyme in a skillet for 7 minutes.
4. Make a pocket in each chiekn breast and stuff each with the msurhoos mixture and cheese.
5. Place these chicken pockets in the baking dish.
6. Bake for 15 minutes in the oven.
7. Serve warm.

Serving Suggestion: Serve the chicken with steaming white rice.

Variation Tip: Add roasted peanuts on top.

Nutritional Information Per Serving:

Calories 301 | Fat 16g |Sodium 189mg | Carbs 32g | Fiber 0.3g | Sugar 0.1g | Protein 28.2g

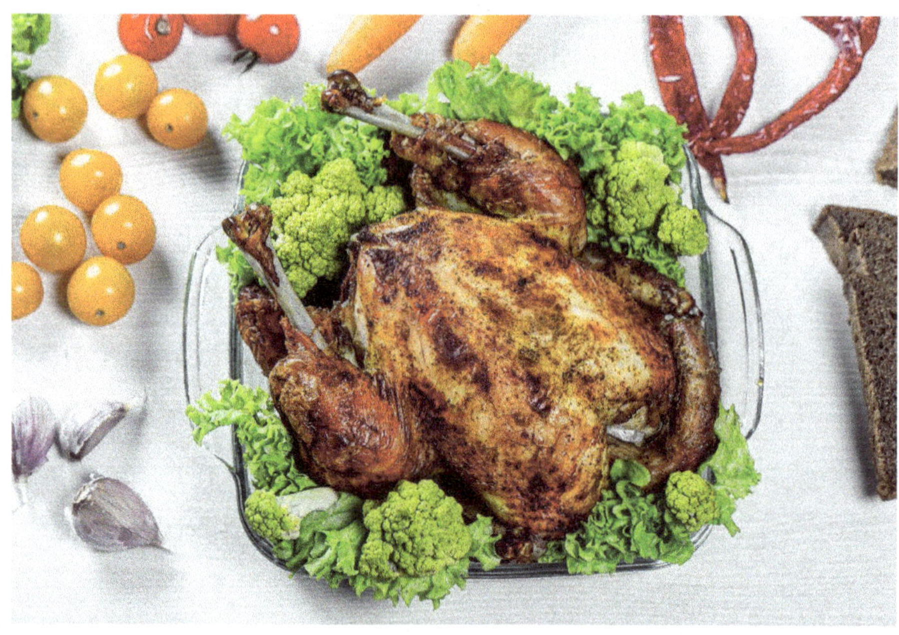

Spinach Mushroom Chicken

Prep Time: 15 minutes.

Cook Time: 43 minutes.

Serves: 4

Ingredients:

- 6 ounces bag raw spinach leaves
- 2 ounces cream cheese
- 2 garlic cloves, minced
- 8 ounces baby bella mushrooms
- 2 teaspoons garlic powder
- 2 teaspoons salt
- 2 teaspoons ground thyme
- 4 chicken breasts
- 4 mozzarella cheese slices

Preparation:

1. At 400 degrees F, preheat your oven.
2. Season chicken with thyme, salt and 1 teaspoon garlic powder.
3. Place this chicken in a casserole dish and bake for 15 minutes in the oven.
4. Saute garlic in a skillet for 1 minute.
5. Stir in spinach and cook for 10 minutes.
6. Add cream cheese then mix well and remove from the heat.

7. Saute mushrooms with thyme, salt, and 1 teaspoon garlic powder in a skillet for 7 minutes.

8. Stir in cream cheese mixture and mix well.

9. Spread this mixture on top of the baked chicken.

10. Drizzle cheese on top and bake another 10 minutes.

11. Serve warm.

Serving Suggestion: Serve the chicken with toasted bread slices.

Variation Tip: Add butter sauce on top of the chicken before cooking.

Nutritional Information Per Serving:

Calories 419 | Fat 13g |Sodium 432mg | Carbs 9.1g | Fiber 3g | Sugar 1g | Protein 21g

Green Lamb Curry

Prep Time: 15 minutes.

Cook Time: 2 hrs. 30 minutes.

Serves: 2

Ingredients:

- 2/3 lb. lean lamb, trimmed and diced
- 2½ tablespoons curry powder
- ½ teaspoons salt
- 1 tablespoon vegetable oil
- 2 onions, sliced
- 4 garlic cloves, chopped
- 1 tablespoon tomato purée
- ½ lb. fresh spinach
- Small bunch of coriander leaves, to serve
- Black pepper, to taste

Preparation:

1. Mix lamb meat with salt, black pepper and curry powder in a bowl.
2. Saute onions with oil in a skillet on medium heat until soft.
3. Stir in lamb and saute until brown.
4. Add garlic, tomato puree and water then cover and cook for 2 hours on medium heat.
5. Remove the lid and cook for 20 minutes.

6.   Stir in spinach and cook for 3 minutes.

7.   Garnish and serve warm.

Serving Suggestion: Serve the curry with white rice.

Variation Tip: Add some kale leaves instead of the spinach

Nutritional Information Per Serving:

Calories 305 | Fat 25g |Sodium 532mg | Carbs 2.3g | Fiber 0.4g | Sugar 2g | Protein 18.3g

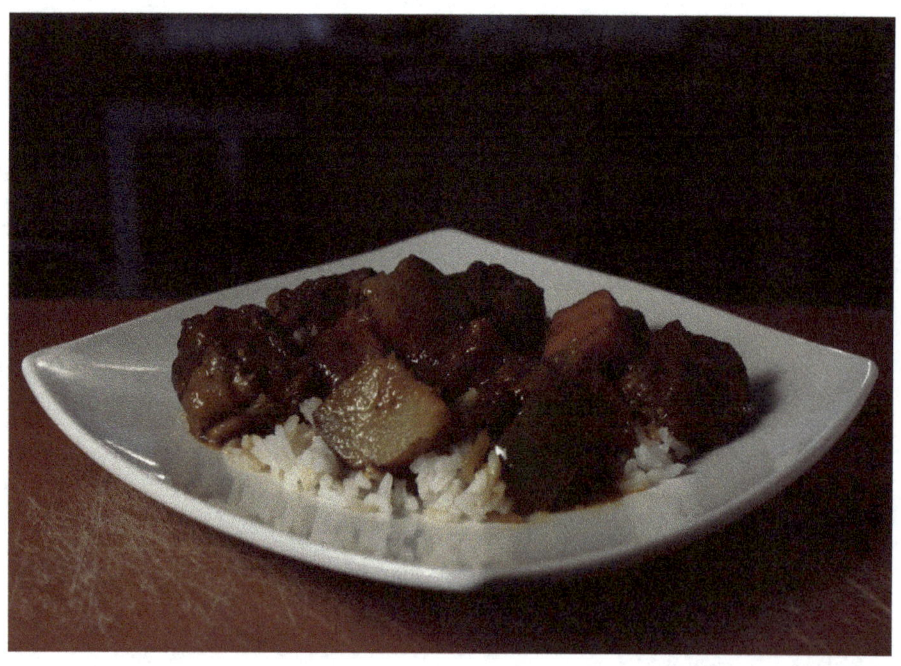

Lamb Pea Curry

Prep Time: 15 minutes.

Cook Time: 22 minutes.

Serves: 2

Ingredients:

- 1 ¼ cups jasmine rice
- Cooking spray oil
- 14 ounces lean lamb medallions
- 5 teaspoons Thai green curry paste
- 1 red onion, sliced
- 14 ounces can creamy coconut evaporated milk
- 2 teaspoons fish sauce
- 1 ½ cups frozen peas
- 14 ounces mix carrot sticks, snow peas, amd broccoli florets

Preparation:

1. Sear the lamb with half of the curry paste and oil in a cooking pan for 2 minutes per side.
2. Cover this lamb and bake for 7 minutes at 400 degrees F.
3. Meanwhile, saute onion with remainig oil and curry paste in a skillet for 1 minute.

4.   Stir in fish sauce and milk then cook for 5 minutes.

5.   Add vegetables and cook for 5 minutes.

6.   Slice the lamb and serve with veggies.

7.   Enjoy.

Serving Suggestion: Serve the curry with toasted bread slices.

Variation Tip: Add crumbled feta cheese on top.

Nutritional Information Per Serving:

Calories 325 | Fat 16g |Sodium 431mg | Carbs 22g | Fiber 1.2g | Sugar 4g | Protein 23g

Lemon Lamb Chops

Prep Time: 15 minutes.

Cook Time: 18 minutes.

Serves: 8

Ingredients:

- Zest of 2 lemons
- 1 tablespoon oregano, chopped
- 1 ¼ teaspoons salt
- Black pepper to taste
- 8 lamb loin chops, trimmed
- 1/4 cup tahini
- ¼ cup nonfat yogurt
- ¼ cup seeded cucumber, diced
- ¼ cup lemon juice
- 2 garlic cloves, minced
- 1 tablespoon fresh parsley, chopped
- 3 tablespoons water
- 2 teaspoons olive oil

Preparation:

1. At 400 degrees F, preheat your ove,
2. Rub the lamb chops with black pepper ¾ teaspoons salt, oregano and lemon zest.
3. Cover and refrigerate these lamb chops for 1 hour.

4. Mix tahini with ½ teaspoons salt, parsley, garlic, lemon juice, cucumber and yogurt in a small bowl.

5. Sear lamb chops with oil in a skillet for 2 minutes per side.

6. Now bake them for 14 mintues in the oven.

7. Pour the tahini sauce on top.

8. Serve warm.

Serving Suggestion: Serve these chops with cauliflower rice.

Variation Tip: Add toasted croutons on top.

Nutritional Information Per Serving:

Calories 425 | Fat 14g |Sodium 411mg | Carbs 44g | Fiber 0.3g | Sugar 1g | Protein 28.3g

Braised Lamb Shanks

Prep Time: 15 minutes.

Cook Time: 2 hr. 30 minutes.

Serves: 4

Ingredients:

- 1 ½ pounds eggplant, peeled
- 4 (12-ounce) lamb shanks, trimmed
- 2 tablespoons ground sumac
- 1 ¼ teaspoons salt
- ½ teaspoon black pepper
- 2 tablespoons olive oil
- 1 green bell pepper, diced
- 1 small onion, diced
- 3 garlic cloves, minced
- 5 plum tomatoes, diced
- 1 cup water
- ½ cup parsley, chopped

Preparation:

1. Rub the lamb shanks with black pepper, salt and 1 tablespoon sumac.
2. Sear lamb with 1 tablespoon oil in a large Dutch oven for 5 minutes per side.
3. Transfer the lamb to a plate.

4. Add remaining 1 tablespoon oil, onion, minced garlic cloves, bell pepper and 1 tablespoon sumac.

5. Saute for 5 minutes then return the lamb to the pot.

6. Stir in tomatoes, water and eggplant then cover and cook on a simmer for 2 hours.

7. Remove the lid and cook for 10 minutes until the gravy thickens.

8. Garnish with parsley and serve warm.

Serving Suggestion: Serve the shanks with sweet potato salad.

Variation Tip: Add chopped green onion to the topping.

Nutritional Information Per Serving:

Calories 425 | Fat 15g |Sodium 345mg | Carbs 12.3g | Fiber 1.4g | Sugar 3g | Protein 23.3g

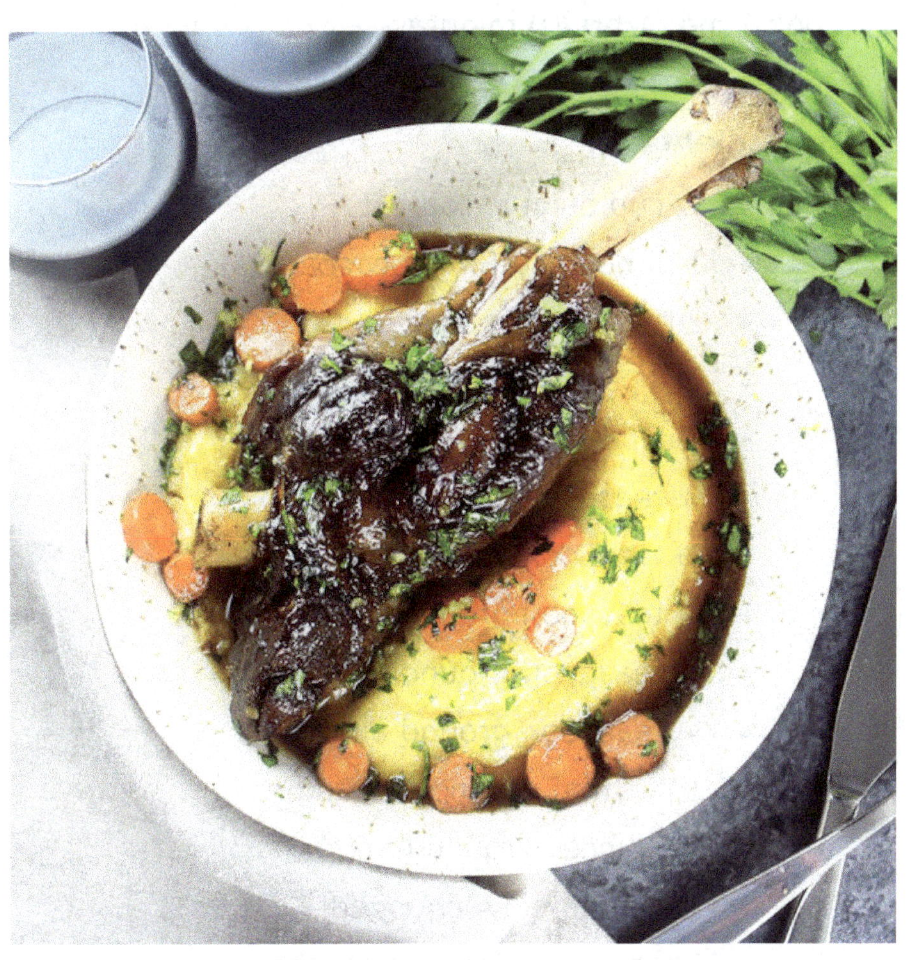

Lamb Cabbage Rolls

Prep Time: 15 minutes.

Cook Time: 1 hr. 10 minutes.

Serves: 8

Ingredients:

- ½ cup bulgur, cooked
- 1 large head Savoy cabbage
- 2 tablespoons olive oil
- 2 cups onion, chopped
- 1 cup leeks, chopped
- ¾ teaspoon salt
- ¾ teaspoon black pepper
- ½ teaspoon ground turmeric
- ¼ teaspoon ground ginger
- ¼ teaspoon ground allspice
- 1 pinch of ground cinnamon
- 12 ounces ground lamb
- ½ cup parsley, chopped
- 2 teaspoons fresh mint, chopped
- 1 large egg, beaten
- ½ cup white wine
- ½ cup chicken broth
- 2 teaspoons lemon zest, grated

- 3 tablespoons lemon juice

Preparation:

1. At 325 degrees F, preheat your oven.
2. Boil cabbage leaves in 2 ½ cups water in a cooking pan and drain.
3. Saute onion and leeks with oil in a skillet for 8 minutes.
4. Add cinnamon, allspice, ginger, turmeric, black pepper and salt then cook for 1 minute.
5. Transfer this mixture to a bowl and add bulgur.
6. Stir in lamb, parsley, mint and egg then mix well.
7. Spread the cabbage leaves o nthe working surface.
8. Divide the lamb filling at the center oeach leave.
9. Wrap the leaves around the filling and place the wrap in a baking dish.
10. Add lemon juice, lemon zest, broth and wine around the cabbage rolls.
11. Cover the dish with a foil sheet and bake for 1 hour in the oven.
12. Serve warm.

Serving Suggestion: Serve the rolls with roasted asparagus.

Variation Tip: Add a drizzle of parmesan cheese on top.

Nutritional Information Per Serving:

 Calories 391 | Fat 5g |Sodium 88mg | Carbs 3g | Fiber 0g | Sugar 0g | Protein 27g

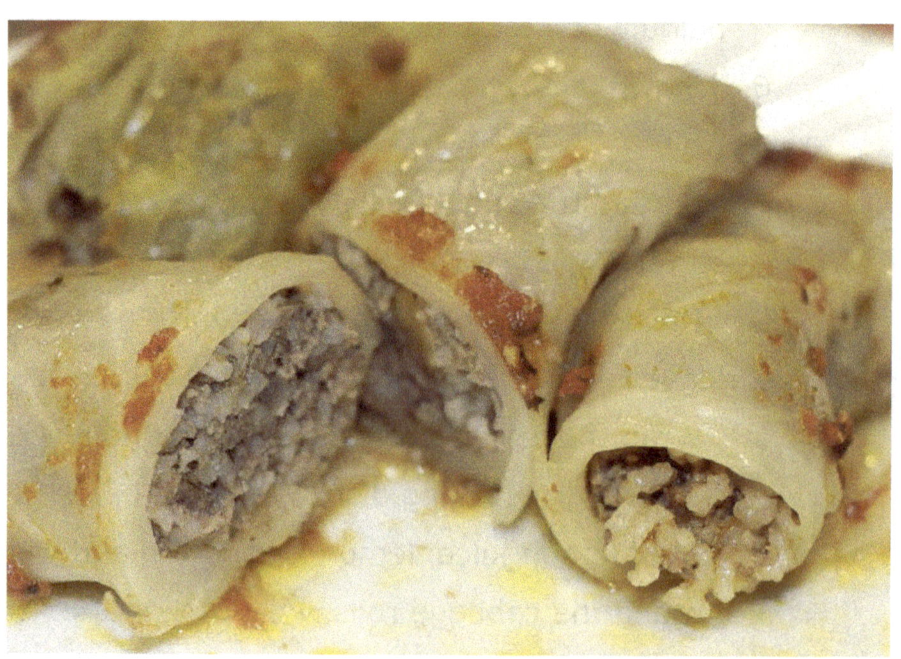

Pork with Caramelized Mushrooms

Prep Time: 15 minutes.

Cook Time: 20 minutes.

Serves: 2

Ingredients:

- 1 lb. lean ground pork
- 8 ounces mushrooms, sliced
- 1 small onion, sliced
- 1 tablespoon garlic, minced
- 1 tablespoon fresh ginger, grated
- 12 ounces bag whole green beans
- 2 tablespoons olive oil
- 1/4 cup water

SAUCE

- 2 tablespoons soy sauce
- 2 tablespoons mirin
- 1 tablespoon rice vinegar
- 2 teaspoons brown sugar
- 1 teaspoon sriracha
- 1 teaspoon dark sesame oil

Preparation:

1. Mix all the sauce ingredients in a small bowl.
2. Saute mushrooms with 1 tablespoon oil in a skillet until soft.

3. Stir in ground pork and saute until brown.

4. Add remaining oil, garlic, ginger, green beans and onion then saute for 2 minutes.

5. Stir in water and cook for another 2 minutes.

6. Pour in the prepared sauce and cook until the liquid is reduced to half.

7. Serve warm.

Serving Suggestion: Serve the pork with cauliflower rice.

Variation Tip: Add a layer of the boiled zucchini noodles to the stir fry.

Nutritional Information Per Serving:

Calories 376 | Fat 21g |Sodium 476mg | Carbs 12g | Fiber 3g | Sugar 4g | Protein 20g

Pepper Taco Bake

Prep Time: 15 minutes.

Cook Time: 30 minutes.

Serves: 4

Ingredients:

- 1 lb. lean ground beef
- 1 tablespoon Phoenix Sunrise Seasoning
- 1 cup vegetable salsa
- 1 ½ lbs fresh bell peppers, quartered
- 1/2 cup cheddar cheese, shredded
- 4 tablespoons sour cream

Preparation:

1. At 350 degrees F, preheat your oven.
2. Mix ground meat with salsa and seasoning in a large bowl.
3. Divide this mixture in the pepper halves and place these peppers in a baking dish.
4. Drizzle cheese on top and bake for 30 minutes in the oven.
5. Garnish with sour cream cheese and serve warm.

Serving Suggestion: Serve the bake with a fresh greens salad.

Variation Tip: Add chopped herbs on top.

Nutritional Information Per Serving:

Calories 487 | Fat 24g |Sodium 686mg | Carbs 17g | Fiber 1g | Sugar 1.2g | Protein 22g

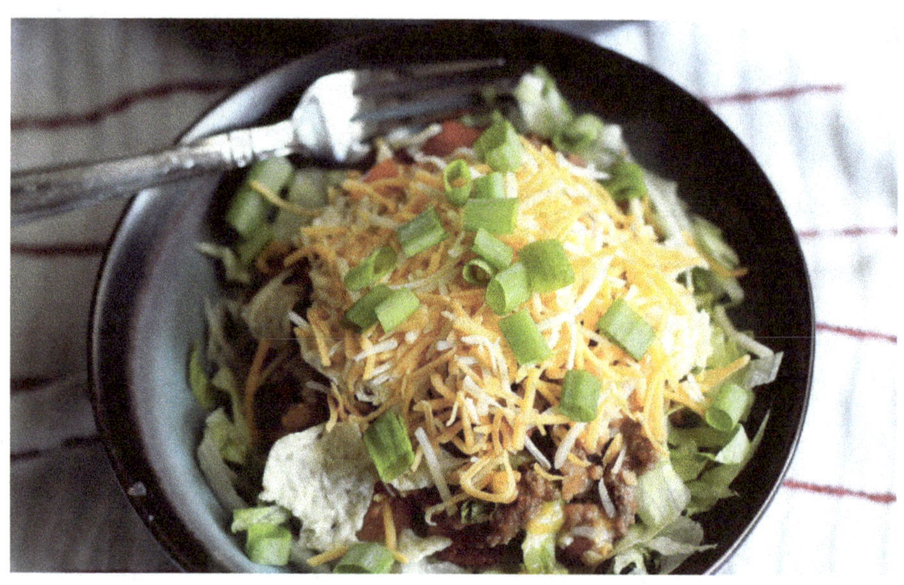

Pan Seared Beef and Mushrooms

Prep Time: 15 minutes.

Cook Time: 17 minutes.

Serves: 4

Ingredients:

- 1 ½ lbs lean beef, cubed
- 1/2 tablespoon Dash of Desperation Seasoning
- Nonstick cooking spray
- 4 cups mushrooms, sliced
- 1 cup beef broth
- 1 ½ teaspoon Garlic Gusto Seasoning

Preparation:

1. Mix beef with seasoning and saute in a skillet with cooking spray for 7 minutes.
2. Add broth and rest of the ingredients and cook or 10 minutes with occasional stirring.
3. Serve warm.

Serving Suggestion: Serve the beef with sweet potato salad.

Variation Tip: Drizzle parmesan cheese on top before serving.

Nutritional Information Per Serving:

Calories 255 | Fat 12g |Sodium 66mg | Carbs 13g | Fiber 2g | Sugar 4g | Protein 22g

Sirloin with Horseradish Sauce

Prep Time: 15 minutes.

Cook Time: 14 minutes

Serves: 2

Ingredients:

- 1 ½ pounds sirloin steaks
- ½ tablesoon dash of desperation seasoning
- 6 tablespoons sour cream
- 3 tablespoons horseradish

Preparation:

1. At medium high heat heat, preheat your grill.
2. Season the steak with Dash seasoning and grill for 7 minutes per side.
3. Mix rest of the ingredients in a bowl.
4. Slice the grilled steak and pour the sauce over steak.
5. Serve warm.

Serving Suggestion: Serve the sirloin with fresh herbs on top.

Variation Tip: Add butter to the meat before serving.

Nutritional Information Per Serving:

Calories 405 | Fat 22.7g |Sodium 227mg | Carbs 26.1g | Fiber 1.4g | Sugar 0.9g | Protein 35.2g

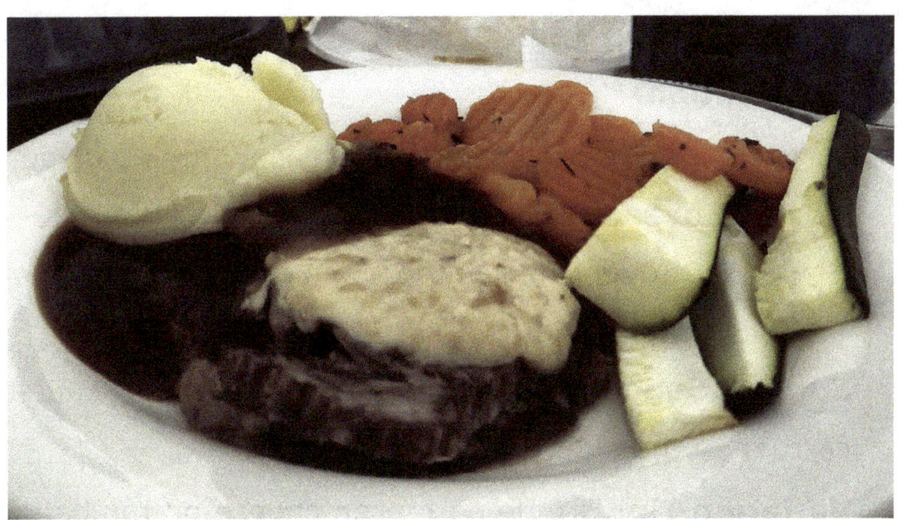

Chipotle Pork Loin

Prep Time: 15 minutes.

 Cook Time: 6 hours.

 Serves: 4

Ingredients:

- 2 pounds boneless pork loin
- 1 tablespoon Garlic and Spring Onion Seasoning
- 1 tablespoon Cinnamon Chipotle Seasoning
- ¼ cup water

Preparation:

1. Add pork loin, water, seasoning and chipotle to a slow cooker.
2. Cover and cook for 6 hours on Low heat.
3. Serve warm.

Serving Suggestion: Serve the pork loin with sautéed carrots on the side.

Variation Tip: Drizzle parmesan cheese on top before serving.

Nutritional Information Per Serving:

Calories 345 | Fat 36g |Sodium 272mg | Carbs 41g | Fiber 0.2g | Sugar 0.1g | Protein 22.5g

Cauliflower Ground Beef Hash

Prep Time: 15 minutes.

Cook Time: 25 minutes.

Serves: 4

Ingredients:

- 16 ounces frozen cauliflower
- 1 lb. lean ground beef
- 2 cups cheddar cheese, shredded
- 1 teaspoon garlic powder
- Salt and black pepper to taste

Preparation:

1. Saute beef in a cooking pan until brown.
2. Stir in garlic, salt, black pepper and cauliflower then cook until soft.
3. Stir in cheddar cheese and cook until the cheese is melted.
4. Serve warm.

Serving Suggestion: Serve the beef hash with sautéed green beans and mashed sweet potatoes.

Variation Tip: Drizzle parmesan cheese on top before cooking.

Nutritional Information Per Serving:

Calories 395 | Fat 9.5g |Sodium 655mg | Carbs 13.4g | Fiber 0.4g | Sugar 0.4g | Protein 28.3g

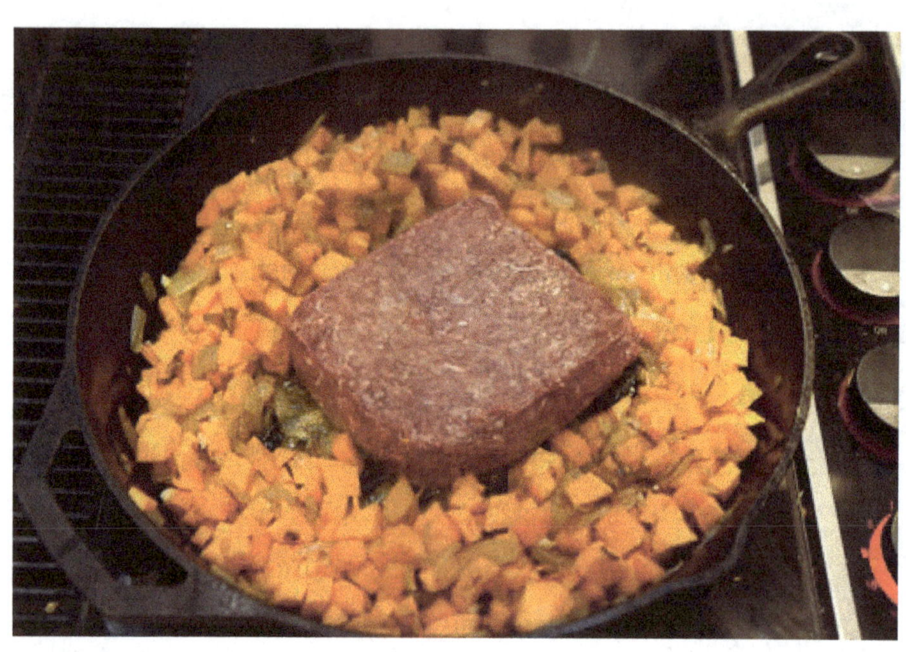

Mojo Marinated Flank Steak

Prep Time: 15 minutes.

Cook Time: 10 minutes.

Serves: 4

Ingredients:

- 2 pounds flank steak
- 2 tablespoons fresh lime juice
- 1 tablespoon garlic Gusto seasoning
- 1 teaspoon ground cumin
- 1/3 cup beef broth
- 1 pinch Dash of Desperation Seasoning

Preparation:

1. Mix beef with remaining ingredients except dash seasoning, in a large bowl.
2. Cover the meat and refrigerate for 1 hour at least.
3. Preheat and grease a grill for cooking.
4. Remove the meat from the marinate and rub with the dash seasoning.
5. Grill the steak for 5 minutes per side.
6. Slice and serve warm.

Serving Suggestion: Serve the steaks with fresh green and mashed sweet potatoes.

Variation Tip: Add zucchini noodles on the side

Nutritional Information Per Serving:

Calories 301 | Fat 5g |Sodium 340mg | Carbs 24.7g |
Fiber 1.2g | Sugar 1.3g | Protein 15.3g

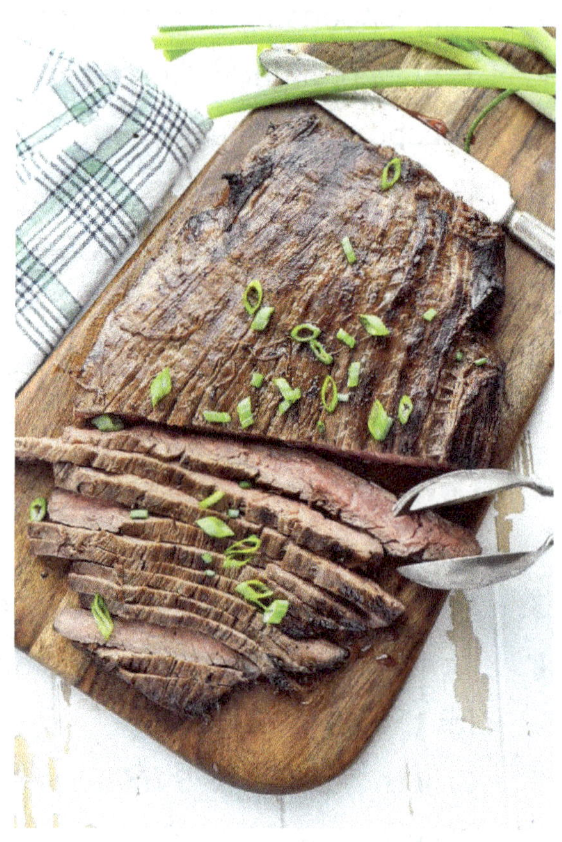

Pork Loin with Tomatoes and Olives

Prep Time: 15 minutes.

Cook Time: 6 hours.

Serves: 4

Ingredients:

- 2 lbs pork tenderloin
- 1 cup chicken broth
- 2 teaspoons Garlic Gusto Seasoning
- 1/2 teaspoon Mediterranean Seasoning
- 10 green olives, sliced
- 1 tablespoon sun dried tomatoes, sliced

Preparation:

1. Add ork and all the ingredients to a crock pot and cover to a cook for 6 hours on Low heat.
2. Slice the meat and serve warm.

Serving Suggestion: Serve the pork with roasted green beans.

Variation Tip: Add sliced black kalamata olives to the pork, if needed.

Nutritional Information Per Serving:

Calories 448 | Fat 23g |Sodium 350mg | Carbs 18g | Fiber 6.3g | Sugar 1g | Protein 40.3g

Pork Tenderloins with Mushrooms

Prep Time: 15 minutes.

Cook Time: 32 minutes.

Serves: 6

Ingredients:

- Cooking spray
- 1 teaspoon dash seasoning
- 1 1/2 lbs pork tenderloin
- 6 cups portobello mushrooms, chopped
- 1/2 cup chicken broth
- 1 tablespoon garlic gusto
- Fresh parsley for garnish

Preparation:

1. At 400 degrees F, preheat your oven.
2. Rub the seasoning over the tenderloin.
3. Sear the tenderloin in a skillet, greased with cooking spray, for 3 minutes per side.
4. Trasnfer the seared pork to a plate.
5. Add rest of the ingredients to the same skillet and cook for 1 minute.
6. Return the pork tenderloin to the skillet and bake for 25 minutes.
7. Slice the pork and serve warm.

Serving Suggestion: Serve the pork with toasted bread slices.

Variation Tip: Replace mushrooms with chopped sweet potatoes.

Nutritional Information Per Serving:

Calories 309 | Fat 25g |Sodium 463mg | Cars 9.9g | Fiber 0.3g | Sugar 0.3g | Protein 28g

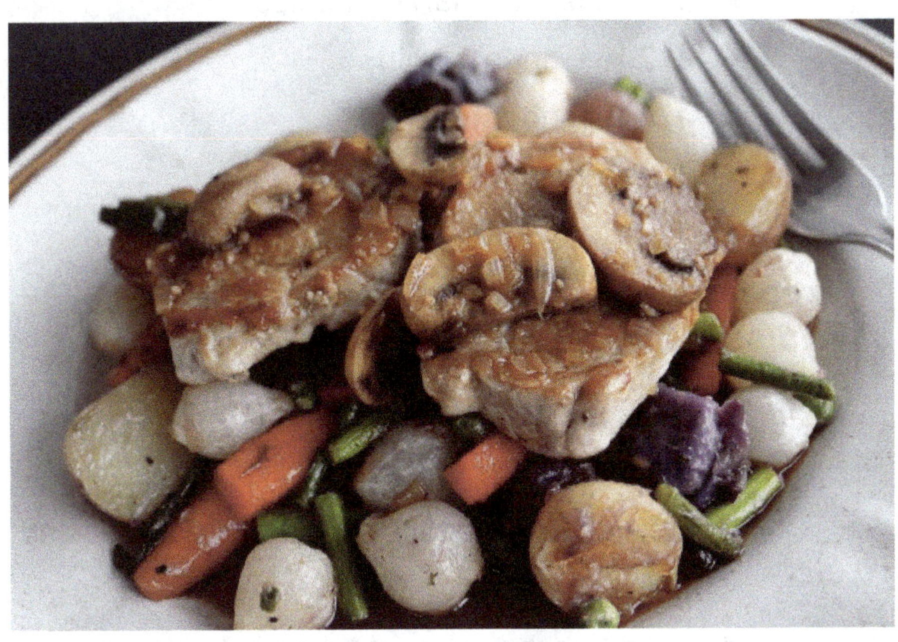

Herb Roasted Tenderloin

Prep Time: 15 minutes.

Cook Time: 60 minutes.

Serves: 8

Ingredients:

- 4 lbs pork tenderloin, lean
- 2 teaspoons black pepper
- 4 tablespoons parmesan cheese, grated
- 2 tablespoons fresh rosemary
- 1 tablespoon fresh thyme
- 1/2 teaspoon garlic, minced
- 1/2 teaspoon cumin
- 1/8 teaspoon salt
- 1 small onion, sliced
- 1/2 cup water

Preparation:

1. At 350 degrees, preheat your oven.
2. Mix cheese with spices in a bowl and rub over the pork.
3. Spread onion slices in a baking sheet and place the pork on top.
4. Add herbs on top and add ½ cup water around the pork.

5. Bake the pork for 1 hour in the preheated oven.

6. Serve warm.

Serving Suggestion: Serve the pork tenderloin with roasted green beans.

Variation Tip: Add paprika for more spice.

Nutritional Information Per Serving:

Calories 537 | Fat 20g |Sodium 719mg | Carbs 25.1g | Fiber 0.9g | Sugar 1.4g | Protein 37.8g

Shrimp Salad

Prep Time: 15 minutes.

Cook Time: 17 minutes.

Serves: 2

Ingredients:

- 2 tablespoons olive oil
- 1/3 cup red onion, chopped
- 3 cups broccoli slaw
- 3 cups broccoli florets
- 1/2 teaspoon salt
- 2 garlic cloves, minced
- 1/2 pound shrimp, peeled and deveined
- 1 teaspoon lime juice
- Green onions, chopped, for garnish
- Cilantro, chopped
- Sriracha and red pepper flakes, for garnish

Sesame almond dressing:

- 2 tablespoons almond butter
- 2 tablespoons water
- 1 tablespoon sesame oil
- 1 tablespoon tamari
- 1 tablespoon maple syrup
- 1 teaspoon lime juice
- 1 teaspoon ginger, minced

- 1 clove minced garlic
- 1 teaspoon sriracha sauce
- 1/4 teaspoon black pepper

Preparation:

1. Mix all the sesame almond dressing in a bowl.
2. Saute onion with oil in a skillet for 5 minutes.
3. Stir in broccoli slaw and florest then saute for 7 minutes.
4. Add black pepper and salt then transfer to a plate.
5. Add minced garlic, shrimp, lime juice and more oil to the same skillet.
6. Saute for 5 minutes then transfer the shrimp to the broccoli.
7. Pour the sesame dressing on top and garnish with cilantro and green onions.
8. Serve warm.

Serving Suggestion: Serve the shrimp salad with cauliflower rice risotto.

Variation Tip: Add paprika for more spice.

Nutritional Information Per Serving:

Calories 212 | Fat 9g |Sodium 353mg | Carbs 8g | Fiber 3g | Sugar 4g | Protein 25g

Salmon Chowder

Prep Time: 15 minutes.

Cook Time: 20 minutes.

Serves: 6

Ingredients:

- 3 tablespoons olive oil
- 1 onion, diced
- 1 small fennel bulb, diced
- 1 cup celery, sliced
- 4 garlic cloves, chopped
- 1 teaspoon fennel seeds
- 1/2 teaspoon thyme
- 1/2 teaspoon smoked paprika
- 1/3 cup vermouth
- 3 cups fish stock
- 3/4 lb baby potatoes, sliced
- 1 teaspoon salt
- 1 bay leaf
- 1 lb salmon, skinless, diced
- 2 cups almond milk

Preparation:

1. lery, fennel, and onion wit Sauté ceh oil in a skillet for 6 minutes.
2. Stir in thyme, fennel seeds and garlic then saute for 2 minutes.
3. Add smoked paprika and vermouth then cook for 2 minutes.
4. Stir in salt, stock, bay, thyme, and potatoes then cook for 10 minutes on a simmer.
5. Stir in salmon bones, salt and milk then cook for 2 minutes.
6. Garnish with lemon wedges, fennel frongs and dill.
7. Serve warm.

Serving Suggestion: Serve the chowder with zucchini noodles.

Variation Tip: Add mixed chopped herbs and lemon zest to the chowder.

Nutritional Information Per Serving:

Calories 376 | Fat 17g |Sodium 1127mg | Carbs 24g | Fiber 1g | Sugar 3g | Protein 29g

Halibut with Zucchini Noodles

Prep Time: 15 minutes.

Cook Time: 17 minutes.

Serves: 8

Ingredients:

- 8 (10 ounces) halibut
- 1 garlic clove, smashed
- 2 tablespoons olive oil
- Salt and black pepper to taste

Noodles:

- 1 tablespoon olive oil
- 1 shallot, sliced
- 3 garlic cloves, chopped
- 16 ounces zucchini noodles
- Salt and black pepper to taste
- 2 teaspoons lemon zest
- ½ cup Italian parsley, chopped
- 1 tablespoon lemon juice

Preparation:

1. At 375 degrees F, preheat your oven.
2. Saute garlic with oil in a skillet over medium heat for 30 seconds.
3. Rub the black pepper and salt over the fish.

4. Sear this fish in the skillet for 6 minutes per side.

5. Transfer this fish to a plate and keep it aside.

6. Stir zucchini, black pepper and salt then saute for 4 minutes.

7. Stir in parsley, lemon zest and lemon juice.

8. Serve the zucchini noodles with fish on top.

9. Enjoy.

Serving Suggestion: Serve the noodles with fresh greens on the side.

Variation Tip: Roll the fish in breadcrumbs for a crispy touch.

Nutritional Information Per Serving:

Calories 457 | Fat 19g |Sodium 557mg | Carbs 19g | Fiber 1.8g | Sugar 1.2g | Protein 32.5g

Poached Mahi Mahi

Prep Time: 15 minutes.

Cook Time: 31 minutes.

Serves: 4

Ingredients:

- 4 (4-ounces) boneless mahi mahi fillets
- 1/4 teaspoon salt
- 1 cup olive oil
- 1 lb asparagus, trimmed
- 3 tablespoons olive oil
- 1 yellow onion, chopped
- 1/4 teaspoon black pepper
- 1 pinch red pepper glakes
- 10 green olives, pitted and chopped
- 1 small head garlic, minced
- 1 cup jarred roasted red peppers, chopped
- 2 tablespoons capers, drained, chopped
- 1/2 cup dry white wine
- 1/2 cup fresh basil, chopped
- 1 tablespoon fresh lemon juice
- Lemon wedges for serving

Preparation:

1. At 250 degrees F, preheat your oven.
2. Rub the fish with salt and keep it aside.

3. Add oil and fish to a skillet and sear for 3 minutes per side.

4. Bake this for 15 minutes then cover and keep it warm.

5. Saute onions with black pepper, pepper flakes and oil in a skillet for 4 minutes.

6. Stir in red pepper, capers, garlic and olives then cook for 2 minutes.

7. Add wine and cook the mixture for 3 minutes on a simmer.

8. Stir in asparagus tips and cook for 1 minute.

9. Add lemon juice, parsley and basil then over the fish.

10. Garnish with lemon wedges.

11. Serve warm.

Serving Suggestion: Serve the fish with cauliflower rice.

Variation Tip: Replace mahi mahi with codfish if needed.

Nutritional Information Per Serving:

Calories 392 | Fat 16g |Sodium 466mg | Carbs 3.9g | Fiber 0.9g | Sugar 0.6g | Protein 48g

Creamy Scallops

Prep Time: 15 minutes.

Cook Time: 9 minutes.

Serves: 3

Ingredients:

- 2 tablespoons olive oil
- 1 ¼ pounds scallops
- 2 tablespoons unsalted butter
- 5 garlic cloves, minced
- Salt and black pepper to taste
- 1/4 cup dry white wine
- 1 cup heavy cream
- 1 tablespoon lemon juice
- 1/4 cup parsley, chopped

Preparation:

1. Sear the scallops in a skillet with oil for 3 minutes per side.
2. Season them with black pepper and salt then transfer to a plate.
3. Saute garlic with 2 tablespoons butter in a skillet for 1 minute.
4. Stir in wine and cook for 2 minutes then add cream.

5. Cook this mixture until mixture thickens then add lemon juice.

6. Return the scallops to the skillet and garnish with parsley.

7. Serve warm.

Serving Suggestion: Serve the scallops with cauliflower salad.

Variation Tip: Add some cream cheese to the scallops.

Nutritional Information Per Serving:

Calories 316 | Fat 22g |Sodium 356mg | Carbs 7g | Fiber 2.4g | Sugar 5g | Protein 18g

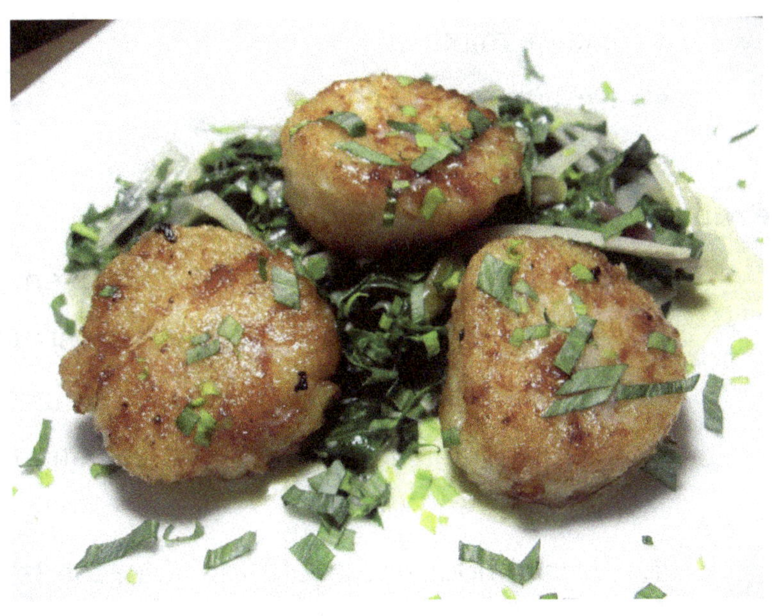

Tuna Broccoli Mornay

Prep Time: 15 minutes.

Cook Time: 30 minutes.

Serves: 4

Ingredients:

- 1 x ½ lb. can Tuna in springwater, drained
- 3 oz. spiral pasta
- 1 head broccoli, florets
- 3 ½ ounce baby spinach leaves, washed
- 1 onion, diced
- 1 ounce butter
- 3 tablespoons flour
- Salt and black pepper, to taste
- 2 cups milk
- 1¼ cup grated cheese
- ¼ cup breadcrumbs

Preparation:

1. At 360 degrees F, preheat your oven.
2. Boil pasta as per the package's instructions then drain and keep it aside.
3. Sauté onion with butter in a cooking pan until sfot.
4. Stir in flour and sauté for 30 seconds.

5.   Add milk, mix well and cook until the mixture thickens.

6.   Add spinach and cook until the leaves are wilted.

7.   Stir in 1 cup grated cheese, broccoli, tuna and black pepper.

8.   Spread this mixture in a casserole dish and spread remaining cheese and breadcrumbs on top.

9.   Bake for 25 minutes in the preheated oven.

10. Serve warm.

Serving Suggestion: Serve the mornay with sautéed vegetables.

Variation Tip: Add canned corn to the mornay.

Nutritional Information Per Serving:

Calories 258 | Fat 9g |Sodium 994mg | Carbs 1g | Fiber 0.4g | Sugar 3g | Protein 16g

Seared Scallops

Prep Time: 15 minutes.

Cook Time: 6 minutes.

Serves: 4

Ingredients:

- 1 lb. large scallops
- Salt, to taste
- Black pepper, to taste
- 1 tablespoon olive oil
- 2 tablespoons butter
- 2 tablespoons parsley, chopped
- Lemon wedges, for serving

Preparation:

1. Season all the scallops with salt, balck pepper, and oil.
2. Melt butter and sear the scallops in a skillet for 3 minutes per side.
3. Drizzle parsley on top and garnish with lemon wedges.
4. Serve warm.

Serving Suggestion: Serve the scallops with lemon slices on top.

Variation Tip: Use white pepper for a change of flavor.

Nutritional Information Per Serving:

Calories 378 | Fat 21g |Sodium 146mg | Carbs 7.1g |
Fiber 0.1g | Sugar 0.4g | Protein 23g

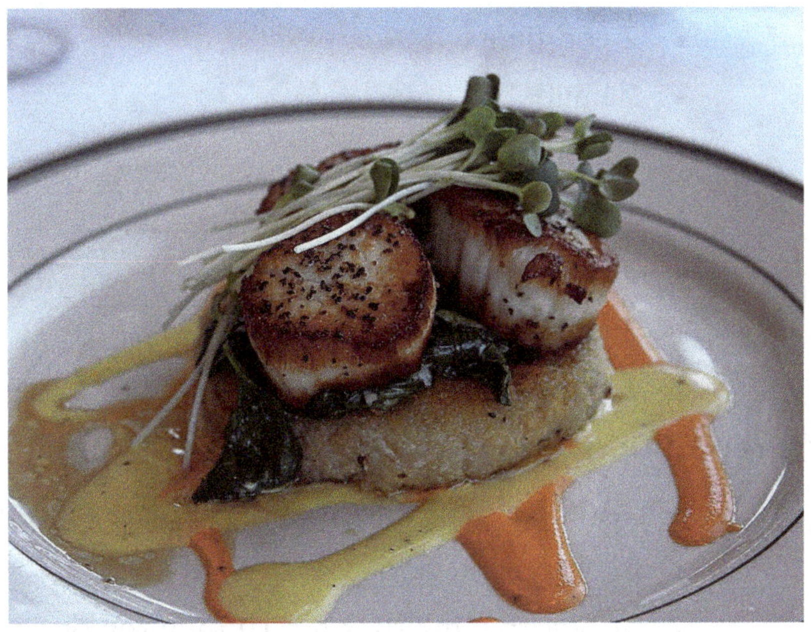

Thai Green Curry

Prep Time: 15 minutes.

Cook Time: 10 minutes.

Serves: 2

Ingredients:

- Fish
- 2 cod fillets
- 2 halibut fillets
- 2 snapper fillets
- 1 lemon
- 2 cups coconut milk
- 3 ounces baby spinach
- 2 ounces carrots, shredded

Preparation:

1. Add coconut milk and rest of the ingredients to a cooking pot.
2. Cook this mixture for 10 minutes on medium heat.
3. Serve warm.

Serving Suggestion: Serve the curry with white rice.

Variation Tip: Drizzle cheese on top for a rich taste.

Calories 351 | Fat 4g |Sodium 236mg | Carbs 19.1g | Fiber 0.3g | Sugar 0.1g | Protein 36g

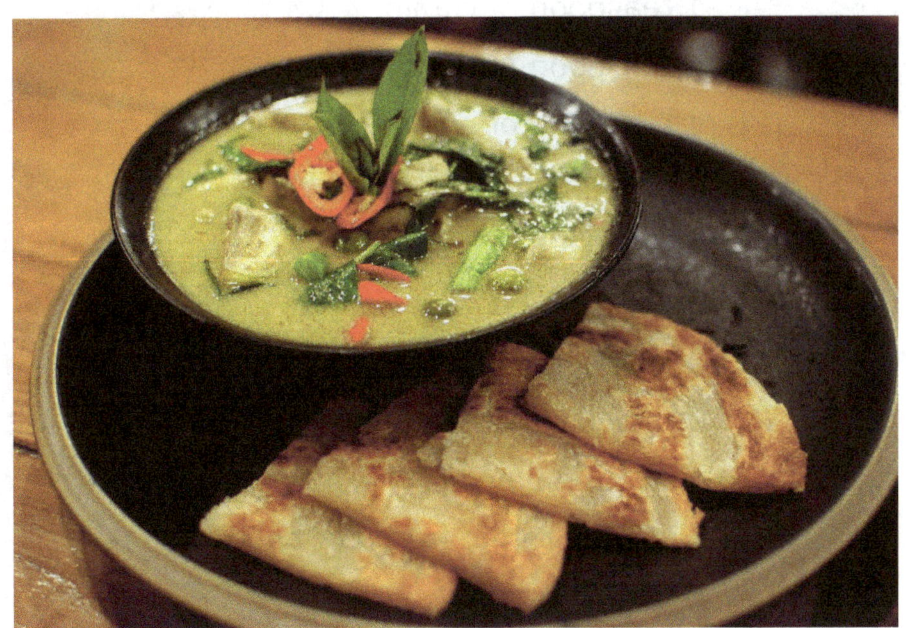

Grilled salmon with Avocado Salsa

Prep Time: 15 minutes.

Cook Time: 10 minutes.

Serves: 4

Ingredients:

- 2 lbs. salmon, cut into 4 fillets
- 1 tablespoon of olive oil
- 1 teaspoon of salt
- 1 teaspoon of cumin
- 1 teaspoon of paprika
- 1 teaspoon of onion
- 1/2 teaspoon chili spices
- 1 teaspoon black pepper

Salsa:

- 1 avocado chopped
- ½ small red onion, sliced
- Juice of 2 limes
- 1 tablespoon of fresh coriander
- Salt, to taste

Preparation:

1. Mix all the spices in a bowl and rub over the salmon fillets along with olive oil.

2. Grill the salmon fillet for 5 minutes per side in a preheated grill.

3.   Chopped avocados with rest of the ingredients in a bowl.

4.   Serve the grilled fish with avocado mash on top.

5.   Enjoy.

Serving Suggestion: Serve the salmon with sweet potato salad.

Variation Tip: Add some chopped bell pepper to the meal.

Nutritional Information Per Serving:

Calories 378 | Fat 7g |Sodium 316mg | Carbs 16.2g | Fiber 0.3g | Sugar 0.3g | Protein 26g

Lemon Garlic Cod with Tomatoes

Prep Time: 15 minutes.

Cook Time: 45 minutes.

Serves: 2

Ingredients:

- 1 ½ pounds cod
- 2 pints cherry tomatoes
- 2 tablespoons olive oil
- 1 teaspoon salt
- 3 garlic cloves, sliced
- 1 tablespoon fresh sage, chopped
- 2 lemons, sliced
- 2 tablespoons capers, for garnish

Preparation:

1. At 325 degrees F, preheat your oven.
2. Place cod in a greased 9x13 inches baking dish.
3. Add tomatoes, olive oil, garlic, sage, lemon and salt on top of the cod.
4. Bake the cod for 45 minutes in the oven.
5. Garnish with capers then serve warm.

Serving Suggestion: Serve the cod with roasted broccoli florets.

Variation Tip: Drizzle lemon zest on top before cooking.

Nutritional Information Per Serving:

 Calories 415 | Fat 15g |Sodium 634mg | Carbs 14.3g | Fiber 1.4g | Sugar 1g | Protein 23.3g

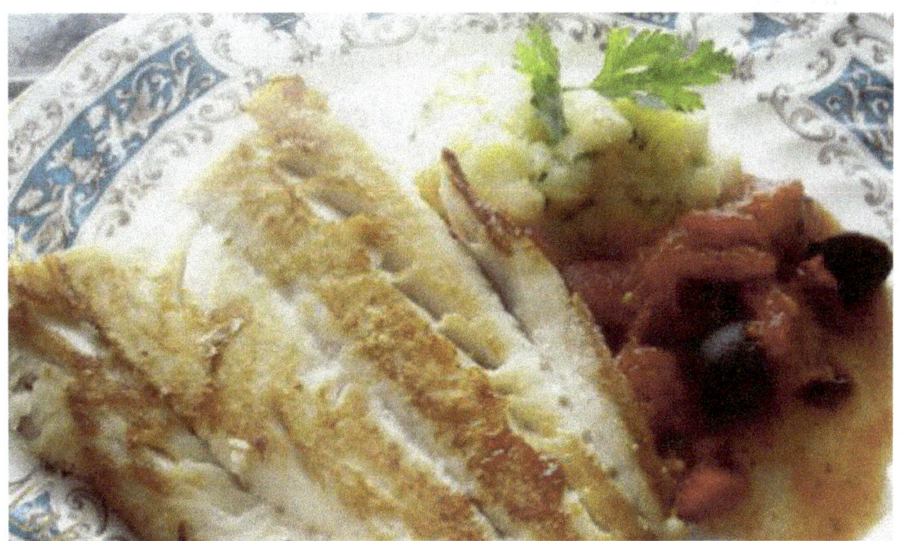

Shrimp Pineapple

Prep Time: 15 minutes.

Cook Time: 15 minutes.

Serves: 4

Ingredients:

- 1 cup pineapple, chopped
- 1lb raw jumbo shrimp
- 1 ½ tablespoons arrowroot starch
- 2 tablespoons avocado oil

Sauce

- 1 tablespoon ginger, minced
- 2/3 cup pineapple juice
- 1 tablespoon garlic, minced
- 3 tablespoon sriracha
- 1 tablespoon soy sauce
- 2 teaspoons arrowroot starch
- 1 tablespoon garlic, minced
- 1 tablespoon honey
- 1/3 cup bell pepper, diced

Garnish

- Fresh green onion
- Sesame seeds
- Fresh limen

Preparation:

1. Mix all the sauce ingredients in a bowl and keep it aside.
2. Toss shrimp with arrowroot in a bowl and shake off the excess.
3. Set a skillet with olive oil over medium heat.
4. Stir in pineapple chunks and cook for 5 minutes.
5. Transfer to a plate and keep them aside.
6. Saute shrimp with avocado oil in the same skillet for 8 minutes.
7. Stir in bell peppers then saute for 1 minute.
8. Add prepared sauce and mix well.
9. Stir in pineapple juice and chunks.
10. Cook for 30 seconds then serve warm.

Serving Suggestion: Serve these shrimps with boiled white rice.

Variation Tip: Add garlic salt to the seasoning for more taste.

Nutritional Information Per Serving:

Calories 251 | Fat 17g |Sodium 723mg | Carbs 21g | Fiber 2.5g | Sugar 2g | Protein 7.3g

Fish Green Curry

Prep Time: 15 minutes.

Cook Time: 13 minutes.

Serves: 4

Ingredients:

- 1 (15-ounce can) coconut milk
- 2 tablespoons green curry paste
- 1 (1-inch) nub fresh ginger, peeled and grated
- 2 tablespoons lime juice
- 2 tablespoons fish sauce
- 1 crown broccoli, chopped
- 2 cups green beans, chopped
- 1 zucchini squash, chopped
- 2 pounds white fish
- Salt, to taste

Serving

- Coconut milk yogurt
- Chives

Preparation:

1. Add coconut milk, lime juice, fish sauce, ginger, and curry paste to a cooking pot and cook to a boil.

2. Stir in green beans and broccoli and cook for 3 minutes.

3.   Stir fish and zucchnini, cover and cook for 10 minutes.

4.   Serve warm.

Serving Suggestion: Serve the fish curry with cauliflower rice.

Variation Tip: Add olives or sliced mushrooms to the fish.

Nutritional Information Per Serving:

Calories 246 | Fat 15g |Sodium 220mg | Carbs 40.3g | Fiber 2.4g | Sugar 1.2g | Protein 12.4g

Vegan Meatballs

Prep Time: 20 minutes.

Cook Time: 48 minutes.

Serves: 4

Ingredients:

- 1 cup cooked quinoa
- 1 (15-ounce) can black beans
- 2 tablespoons water
- 3 garlic cloves, minced
- 1/2 cup shallot, diced
- 1/4 teaspoon salt
- 2 1/2 teaspoon fresh oregano
- 1/2 teaspoon red pepper flake
- 1/2 teaspoon fennel seeds
- 1/2 cup vegan parmesan cheese, shredded
- 2 tablespoons tomato paste
- 3 tablespoons fresh basil, chopped
- 2 tablespoons Worcestershire sauce

Preparation:

1. At 350 degrees F, preheat your oven.
2. Spread the beans in a baking sheet and bake for 15 minutes.
3. Meanwhile, sauté garlic, shallots and water to a skillet for 3 minutes.

4. Transfer to the food processor along with fennel, red pepper flakes, baked beans, oregano and salt.
5. Blend these ingredients just until incorporated.
6. Stir in quinoa, and rest of the ingredients then mix evenly.
7. Make golf-ball sized meatballs out of this mixture.
8. Spread these meatballs in a grease baking sheet and bake for 20-30 minutes until brown.
9. Flip the meatballs once cooked half way through.
10. Serve warm.

Serving Suggestion: Serve the meatballs with pita bread and chili sauce.

Variation Tip: Add chopped mushrooms to the batter as well.

Nutritional Information Per Serving:

Calories 338 | Fat 24g |Sodium 620mg | Carbs 58.3g | Fiber 2.4g | Sugar 1.2g | Protein 5.4g

Minestrone Soup

Prep Time: 15 minutes.

Cook Time: 40 minutes.

Serves: 6

Ingredients:

- 1 yellow onion, diced
- 3 garlic cloves, minced
- 1 carrot peeled and diced
- 4 celery stalks, diced
- 4 cups vegetable broth
- 1 (15-ounces) can of tomato juice
- 1 (15-ounces) can of diced tomatoes
- 8 ounces elbow pasta
- 1 (15ounces) can of red kidney beans rinsed and drained
- 1 (15ounces) can of white beans
- 2 handfuls baby spinach, chopped
- 1 teaspoon coriander
- 1 teaspoon oregano
- 1 teaspoon black pepper
- 1 teaspoon basil
- 1 teaspoon paprika
- Salt to taste
- Chopped parsley for garnish

Preparation:

1.   Add carrot, garlic, celery, onion and vegetable broth in a cooking pot and cook for 20 minutes on a simmer.
2.   Stir in rest of the ingredients and cook for 20 minutes.
3.   Garnish with parsley.
4.   Serve warm.

Serving Suggestion: Serve the soup with avocado salad.

Variation Tip: Add chopped mushrooms to the soup as well.

Nutritional Information Per Serving:

Calories 393 | Fat 3g |Sodium 510mg | Carbs 12g | Fiber 3g | Sugar 4g | Protein 4g

Tofu Fried Rice

Prep Time: 10 minutes.

Cook Time: 13 minutes.

Serves: 4

Ingredients:

- 1 package baked tofu
- 4 cup cauliflower rice
- 1 cup frozen peas
- 1 cup carrots, shredded
- 1 teaspoon onion powder
- 1 teaspoon garlic powder
- 1/2 cup soy sauce
- 1/4 cup scallions, chopped
- Salt and black pepper to taste

Preparation:

1. Saue tofu with peas, carrots, garlic powder, soy sauce, scallions, black pepper and salt in a cooking pan for 10 minutes.
2. Stir in cauliflower rice and mix well.
3. Cover and cook for 3 minutes on medium heat.
4. Serve warm.

Serving Suggestion: Serve the rice with kale salad.

Variation Tip: Add boiled couscous to the mixture.

Nutritional Information Per Serving:

 Calories 378 | Fat 3.8g |Sodium 620mg | Carbs 13.3g |
Fiber 2.4g | Sugar 1.2g | Protein 5.4g

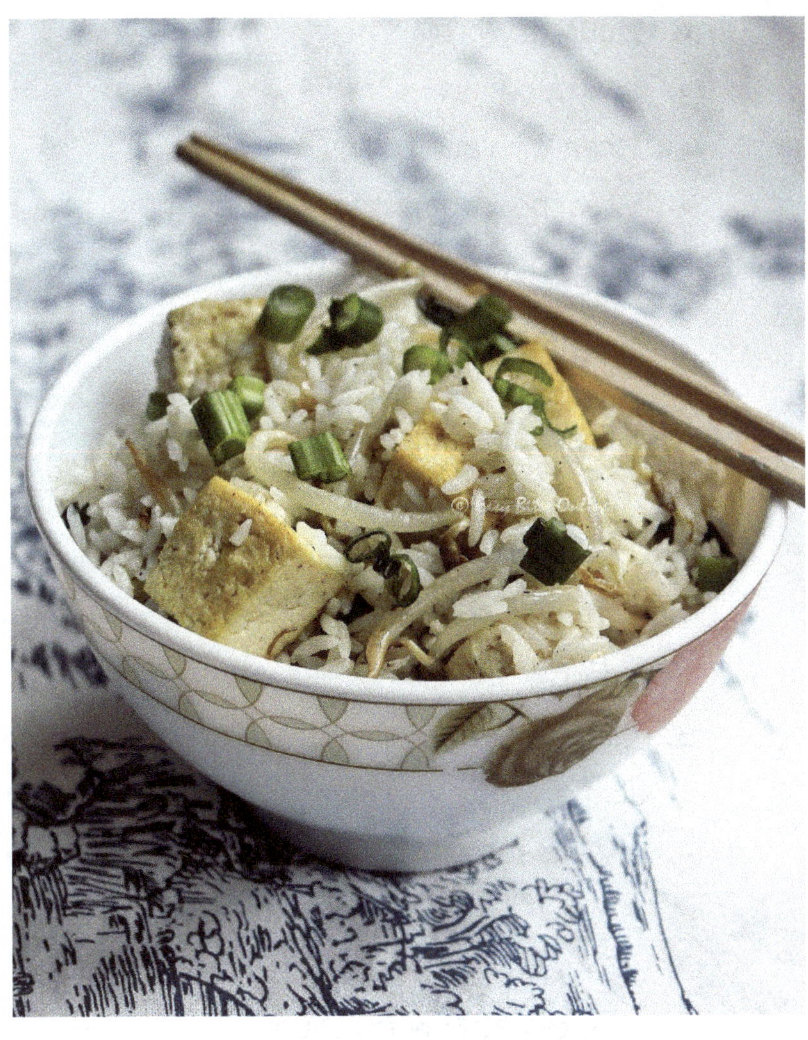

Rice and Beans

Prep Time: 15 minutes.

Cook Time: 22 minutes.

Serves: 4

Ingredients:

- 1 cup dry brown rice
- 1 ½ cup water
- 1 can of black beans
- 1 teaspoon paprika
- 1 teaspoon garlic powder
- 1 teaspoon oregano
- 1 teaspoon cumin
- 1 teaspoon onion powder

Preparation:

1. At 350 degrees F, preheat your oven.
2. Add water and rice to the Pressure Pot's insert.
3. Set a trivet over the rice and place a baking dish on top.
4. Add beans and rest of the ingredients to this bowl.
5. Cover and seal the lid and cook for 22 minutes at Low pressure.

6.   Once done, release all the pressure and remove the lid.

7.   Mix the beans and transfer to a serving plate.

8.   Serve the beans with the rice.

9.   Enjoy.

Serving Suggestion: Serve the beans with the spinach salad.

Variation Tip: Add crispy fried onion on top for better taste.

Nutritional Information Per Serving:

Calories 304 | Fat 31g |Sodium 834mg | Carbs 21.4g | Fiber 0.2g | Sugar 0.3g | Protein 4.6g

Corn Chowder

Prep Time: 15 minutes.

Cook Time: 28 minutes.

Serves: 8

Ingredients:

- 4 cups vegetable broth
- 8 cups corn
- 1 whole yellow onion, diced
- 1 tablespoon chili powder
- 1 teaspoon salt
- 4 cups water
- 1/4 cup nutritional yeast
- 1/4 lime juiced
- 1/4 cup cilantro

Preparation:

1. Add vegetable broth, onion, corn and chili powder to a cooking pot.
2. Cook for 8 minutes with occasional stirring.
3. Remove 1/3 of this cooking mixture and keep it aside.
4. Add water to the rest and cook for 20 minutes on a simmer.
5. Puree the cooked corn soup until smooth.

6.   Stir in lime juice, yeast, and remaining corn mixture.

7.   Serve warm with cilantro on top.

8.   Enjoy.

Serving Suggestion: Serve the chowder with cauliflower salad.

Variation Tip: Top the chowder cheddar cheese with before serving.

Nutritional Information Per Serving:

Calories 341 | Fat 24g |Sodium 547mg | Carbs 36.4g | Fiber 1.2g | Sugar 1g | Protein 10.3g

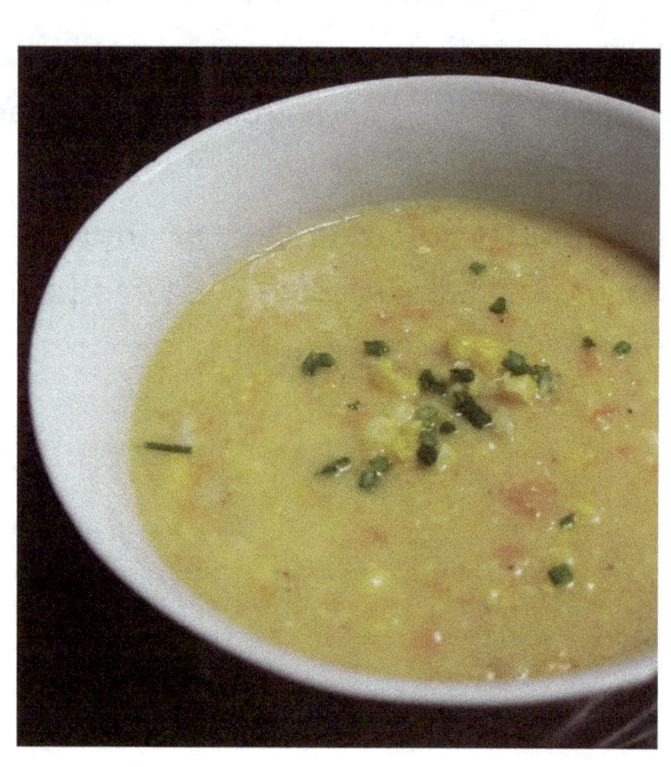

CPSIA information can be obtained
at www.ICGtesting.com
Printed in the USA
BVHW091215230621
610125BV00020B/739